NEW WAY TO GRIEVE

From Grieving to Living:
Getting Unstuck and Finding
the Life That Fits You Now

PAULETTE KRANJAC

NEW WAY TO GRIEVE
ISBN 978-0-578-83192-3
Non-fiction by Paulette Kranjac
Copyright ©2021 by Paulette Kranjac
Published 2021 by Paulette Kranjac
All rights reserved. No part of this publication may be reproduced, stored in a retrieval system, or transmitted in any form or by any means: electronic, mechanical, photocopy, recording, or otherwise, without the prior written permission of the publisher.

New Way to Grieve by Paulette Kranjac is a book for those who have grieved, are grieving, or will be grieving. Of course, this description encompasses almost everyone, and it includes those who are actively on the grieving continuum; from those who are demolished by their loss, to those who would prefer to avoid and deny it.

In her work, Kranjac makes it clear that to be alive is to grieve. However, the essence here is about changing our relationship with grief, almost embracing it as part of the human experience. Utilizing her own bereavement experiences as a foundation while incorporating her own research and training, Kranjac has written a primer for people caught up in, or surely going to be in, the process.

Written from the heart, this work includes a wealth of real-life experiences, some of a very personal nature and other touching vignettes based on the author's interactions with bereaved others. Her in-depth exploration of the bereavement experience provides scores of helpful suggestions and exercises designed to assist anyone going through grief, normalizing thoughts and feelings be they from a place of anger, guilt, denial, despair or whatever.

One important "takeaway" from this work is to acknowledge the gratitude we have for those in our lives right at this very moment and, as much as possible, living life to the fullest and being present to it. For no one knows just when the "bell will toll" for them or for their loved ones. Therefore, without just sitting here and waiting for the other shoe to drop, we might as well be prepared and perhaps just a bit more appreciative.

Lawrence M. Tunis, Ed.D, LMFT

Foreword

Grieving cannot be done on a timeline. However, grief does not need to stop you from living life. Do you feel like something is preventing you from moving forward and you would like to get back to living more fully?

Welcome to *New Way to Grieve*, a book for anyone who wants relief from grief. I wrote this book because I discovered how to do just that.

If you find yourself in any of the descriptions below, you are precisely why I wrote *New Way to Grieve*.

- You have become hopeless about the future and feel that it is enough to just get through your day. Each day seems much the same as the one before.
- You assert the same regrets such as, "If only I had done this, they might be alive. If only they had not done that, they might still be here. I just don't know how I can go on without them!"
- You say things like, "S/he was my everything and I will never find someone else." You may even use that notion to convince yourself that is the reason you cannot move forward.
- Your sadness does not seem to let up.
- You have recurring and upsetting thoughts, worries, guilt, and anger.
- You ponder why things did not work out for you. Or you fear that this is what you must live with for the rest of your life.

Even though sadness can be quite difficult to manage, I discovered a new way to grieve after experiencing 13 deaths in one decade. I am sharing my story so that you do not have to add more pain to your suffering.

The tools I outline in this book are based on my own journey and helped me live a rich life, despite my grief. By reading this book and doing the grief work that I recommend, you can move forward and create a new life.

What is unique about New Way to Grieve?

New Way to Grieve addresses a new ability to experience and express your sadness as the pure grief that it is rather than the 'grief' we seem to endure because of our thoughts about our loved one's death. These thoughts might have us so stuck that we do not participate fully in life. Not just early on in grief, but sometimes for months, years, and even decades we postpone or entirely give up on our dreams and our lives.

This is not your mother's book about grief. It is not an updated version of Elisabeth Kübler-Ross's *'stages of grief.'*

Nor anything like Sheryl Sandberg's *Option B*, or Joan Didion's *The Year of Magical Thinking*. By reading this book you will not be able to discern what stage you are in your grief journey such as anger, denial, or bargaining. This book does not suggest that you keep yourself busy, accept your lot in life, or deal with the cards you are dealt.

New Way to Grieve is based on everything useful that I learned during my journey of plentiful, substantial loss and radical, sudden loss: 12 people in the previous ten years, and then Tom, my husband who I was with for 43.5 years, died suddenly.

Foreword

The idea of separating our circumstances from our thoughts is not my original idea. I pay homage to Werner Erhard, founder of *est* and source of Landmark Worldwide. This transformational work played a key role in my being able to separate this tragedy from all the tales I might have attached to it had I not done this work. It also allowed me to see that by forgiving the past and by becoming aware of the words I used to describe my situation, I could move forward into a created future.

Among many things, New Way to Grieve will:

- Recommend useful ways to manage your well-being for the most productive, long-term benefits.
- Take you through the process of separating your pure sadness from the secondary thoughts that leave you trapped.
- Provide you with exercises to feel and express anger toward your loved one so that you can forgive and feel the freedom to dream about your life.
- Walk you through the process of forgiving yourself so you feel like you deserve to take steps to accomplish your dreams.
- Offer tools to surf the waves of grief so you can set yourself up in the most powerful way as you anticipate and mitigate the triggers of everyday life.
- Suggest how to keep connected in all relationships so that you have peace, love, and a future of connection in your life both when your loved one is dying and after.
- Move you toward finding your purpose, perhaps honoring your loved one in inspiring ways and through discovering what truly fits you now.

I have formulated this book from significant and life-altering experiences. These include exposure to, and knowledge gained from a wide variety of educational, growth-oriented, and spiritual learning, including but not limited to:

- Master of Arts in psychology, public health courses at CUNY, The Herbert Benson, MD Course in Mind, Body, Medicine at Harvard Medical School.
- Grand rounds and symposiums at The New York Academy of Science, Northwell Health, and Cornell.
- Knowledge gained from my own self-discovery modalities including psychotherapy and psychoanalysis, transformational education, the *est* Training 1978, The Landmark forum, and other Landmark Worldwide courses 2014-2020, Being A Leader and The Effective Exercise of Leadership created by Werner Erhard, Michael C. Jensen, Grief Recovery Method certification achieved in 2017.
- Ten years of a Transcendental Meditation practice with training received by Bob Roth, The David Lynch Foundation.
- Nine years of awareness practice of self and outward-directed compassion, inspired by Romemu, a renewal synagogue in New York City and Rabbi David Ingber.
- A personal commitment to regular exercise for 44 years and a healthy lifestyle for 11 years.
- A fierce can-do passion and resilience inherited from my mom, Sylvia Tunis, who, without means or support, raised three incredible kids as a single mom in the early 1950's – unheard of in a Jewish family.

Will you get value from reading New Way to Grieve?

That is up to you. Throughout the book I share some powerful exercises for you to do.

If you have had enough suffering and feeling stuck, and if you are ready to approach your grief in a new way, take these exercises seriously and do them. Choose a dedicated journal to use and keep it with you as

Foreword

you go through this book. There may be some pain involved in doing this initially, yet once it is expressed, you can begin to achieve peace of mind. It is then that you may be able to fashion a meaningful and enjoyable future filled with new dreams.

Using the tools I share about my own journey through this process, you will be able to experience the pure sadness you have, forgive what happened, and move forward.

Though this may seem an elusive concept right now, I hope this book will help you discover a new ability to dream and to take actions to make your future dreams a reality.

Paulette Kranjac

My personal prepublication note to you regarding the pandemic:

I wrote this book during COVID-19 when there seemed some end in sight. With the uptick and morphing of the virus, despite the fact we have a vaccine, I understand the possibly complex challenges of seeing a creative vista on the horizon and physically going out and about to connect with people.

We do have online access, and we can have personal patience for global health. We have imagination and the ability to dream which I am certain will be sharpened by reading this book. We do not have to allow our grief circumstances to stop us. And we do not have to allow the upholding of COVID-19 safety strategies to stop us either. Thank you.

This book is dedicated to the memory of my late husband, Dr. Thomas Kranjac, my partner for 43½ years who died suddenly on April 30, 2016. It is the culmination of my grief journey and my stand that his life will be for a blessing.

Paulette Kranjac

Contents

Grief Sufferer to Grief Surfer	15
Your Well-Being while Grieving	22
What is Grief?	31
Thoughts and Worries	36
Staying Connected Regardless of Others' Thoughts	43
A Wish List for your Future	49
Anger First, then Forgiving your Loved One	52
Anger, then Forgiving Yourself	65
Freedom to Dream to See what Fits You Now	71
What Doesn't Fit You	78
The Heaven can Wait Phenomenon	85
Honoring Your Loved One	93
Grief and Terminal Illness	98
Sudden Death	104
Creating a Team with your Siblings (even if it seems difficult)	113
Making it through Each Day of the Year	120
Living your Purpose	127
What is Next	130
Acknowledgments	135
About the Author	139
About the Cover Art	141

Grief Sufferer to Grief Surfer

Grief is a matter of the heart and soul. Grieve your loss, allow it in, and spend time with it. Suffering is the optional part.
LOUISE HAY AND DAVID KESSLER

SUDDENLY ALONE AFTER OVER FOUR DECADES with my husband, with a college son to support emotionally and financially, no local family members, and a dozen recent losses, I was dealing with huge sadness, trauma, downsizing, and other issues concerning a death unplanned for.

Three weeks after my husband died, I joined a support group in Manhattan for widows. Immediately I noticed myself offering leadership and comfort to those who had been attending these meetings regularly for six or even nine years. Yikes, nine years, and they are still crying? I did not know much then about recovering from significant and sudden grief, but if they were still reliving their situations almost a decade later, this was not something I wanted to be signing up for. I decided to quit the group.

Then I joined a few widows and widowers' groups on Facebook. I looked to find myself in others' stories. Reading the posts, I wanted to know if my issues were similar to others and how were they functioning during grief.

To my surprise, the common thread of the Facebook posts was "Why me?" or "I am so stuck" or "How can I go on?" What was more disturbing was it became apparent that people were speaking about being stuck for years if not decades, and in fact were asking, "Will this pain ever end?"

One post from a widow was about the emotions evoked when she was invited to join her late husband's family for the holidays. "How could they ask me to join them when I am grieving?" she posted. The widow shared that she was angry and enraged.

I read this and thought, "How fortunate that they *want* to include her, that she is still seen as family even though he died. Can she see that she could also be grateful?" I realized this woman would be furious if the family did NOT ask her to come, yet she was also angry at being asked. I took a breath and posted exactly that.

Within minutes the replies, likes, and positive emojis began coming fast. Some appreciated my being straightforward and some asked me how I gained this insight. Some reached out by messenger and then some phoned. A few became friends.

I saw the unique way that I handled life and grief. And that needed to be shared. I discovered that my mission is to help people participate and move forward in life despite the death of their loved one. I want to help create a world where people do not add more pain to their grief.

Most profoundly, out of this tragedy, I adopted the aspect of making a difference to honor Tom's life. I have committed myself to sharing his life which already was 'for a blessing.'

Grief Sufferer to Grief Surfer

Grief is a matter of the heart and soul. Grieve your loss, allow it in, and spend time with it. Suffering is the optional part.
LOUISE HAY AND DAVID KESSLER

SUDDENLY ALONE AFTER OVER FOUR DECADES with my husband, with a college son to support emotionally and financially, no local family members, and a dozen recent losses, I was dealing with huge sadness, trauma, downsizing, and other issues concerning a death unplanned for.

Three weeks after my husband died, I joined a support group in Manhattan for widows. Immediately I noticed myself offering leadership and comfort to those who had been attending these meetings regularly for six or even nine years. Yikes, nine years, and they are still crying? I did not know much then about recovering from significant and sudden grief, but if they were still reliving their situations almost a decade later, this was not something I wanted to be signing up for. I decided to quit the group.

Then I joined a few widows and widowers' groups on Facebook. I looked to find myself in others' stories. Reading the posts, I wanted to know if my issues were similar to others and how were they functioning during grief.

To my surprise, the common thread of the Facebook posts was "Why me?" or "I am so stuck" or "How can I go on?" What was more disturbing was it became apparent that people were speaking about being stuck for years if not decades, and in fact were asking, "Will this pain ever end?"

One post from a widow was about the emotions evoked when she was invited to join her late husband's family for the holidays. "How could they ask me to join them when I am grieving?" she posted. The widow shared that she was angry and enraged.

I read this and thought, "How fortunate that they *want* to include her, that she is still seen as family even though he died. Can she see that she could also be grateful?" I realized this woman would be furious if the family did NOT ask her to come, yet she was also angry at being asked. I took a breath and posted exactly that.

Within minutes the replies, likes, and positive emojis began coming fast. Some appreciated my being straightforward and some asked me how I gained this insight. Some reached out by messenger and then some phoned. A few became friends.

I saw the unique way that I handled life and grief. And that needed to be shared. I discovered that my mission is to help people participate and move forward in life despite the death of their loved one. I want to help create a world where people do not add more pain to their grief.

Most profoundly, out of this tragedy, I adopted the aspect of making a difference to honor Tom's life. I have committed myself to sharing his life which already was 'for a blessing'.

Grief Sufferer to Grief Surfer

I wrote a poem describing my experience of grief about six weeks after Tom died.

I'm a Grief Surfer

I'm a Grief Surfer riding the waves of a giant ocean
Sometimes there is calm where I am.
The horizon is invigorating because by God, I'm doing it.
From nowhere a huge wave of despair hits.
Memories flow as I think about his touch, his smell, his
    thinking, his words and voice, strength, and passion.
I ride this wave and the pain recedes back to the ocean itself.
Sometimes I think "How am I going to live my life without him?"
This wave is the most robust, the scariest and the one most
    ominous.
I awake in good health. I am blessed with my son and I arise
    with so many amazing purposes in my life.
I am however deeply at sea.
Tom is not beside me, nor will I ever see him again.
For sure I am dreaming this, and I am caught in an awful frame
    within the movie *Groundhog Day*
Overhead this cloud feels just like the day before and the day
    before that.
A baseline of sadness exists for me that is always ready to
    show up.
It comes to me when I am not fully engaged in my life even for
    a second.
It shows up when I pause to think, when I pause to rest, when
    I meditate, in between my work and my work outs and in
    between my care for my daily life.
Grief-isms by others:
    Are you functioning, eating, and sleeping, they ask?
    Are you complete with who you were for each other?

Surround yourself with people who love you only.
Be with what you are going through.
Empower yourself and participate.
Be strong.
Grief is biological and chemical.
It is the brain's way of completing all facets of what occurred.
You need to experience this all out.

I feel the pain freshly when I gaze into the faces of our past.
    I see Tom—even through my dog's cues to me and her non- stop apparent searching for her 'Daddy' around the corners—and across the avenues.
The sea I am riding on holds all the dreams for our future which ended so suddenly.
It holds what was planned, unfulfilled and taken too soon from my husband Tom and from me and my dear son.
I will be on this slick, fast, and narrow, black-colored surfboard for 11 months in these awful seas.[1]
I will manage my well-being and my son's, but not my grief, for grief manages through me.
I will begin to recreate the memory and blessing that my dear Tom was for me and others – the impact of his life and my commitment to carrying the torch for his future memory.
I have endured the grief surf many times but never have I lost my rock and my soulmate nor incurred so sudden a shock.
I stand for sharing what I know to help others not have pain.
    To make others a bit more comfortable, a bit more able to adapt, a bit more resilient, a bit more empowered with resources and perhaps more knowledgeable and thus, perhaps even happier.

---

1 Eleven months in the Jewish calendar after the first thirty days (Shloshim) is what I had thought was the mourning period when I wrote this poem. This applies to loss of a parent. I notate this here for clarification.

> I will keep sharing myself and my grief surfing, not the adventure I had planned for...but it is the one I am currently riding.[2]

Surfing, riding on the waves of grief, reminders, feelings, memories, nuances, intense sadness, and thoughts about your loved one will come up unpredictably – just like that of a large wave rolling up onto the beach from previously calm waters.

I recommend just going with it. Allow yourself to feel the sadness and to cry. Share your sad feelings. The sadness or memory that comes up does not have to throw you into a depression or a funk. More importantly, it does not have to throw you into the thought that something is wrong with you.

The sadness is the pure grief that you are experiencing. It is just sadness. Sometimes deep sadness. Ask your friends to be the listeners in your life right now and to be receptive to hearing your sadness. Allow yourself to go out, to go on, and to greet each new day as best you can.

My husband's sudden death began what seemed to be a very dark, bleak path for me, with no future vista nor solid, close support system in place. First gradually, then more and more, I went out finding an event to attend or an experience in which to engage, exploring life and anything I thought might be of interest.

The point of being a 'grief surfer' is that just because you may be outside of your home, you do need not to feel happy nor be smiley. What is important is living your life despite your thoughts and worries. Allowing your sadness to come up when it surfaces as you live each day enables you to move forward, rebuild life, and even share with

---

2   Poem titled by Sue Kennedy, writer.

others along the way. I found that sharing with others can lead to deep connections.

Tom used to remind me that that life is finite for each of us. And even if someone is dying, we still need to live. When I would come home from the hospital for the sixth time each day looking after my mother, Tom would say, "Remember for whom the bell tolls? It tolls for thee."

Yes, surfers ride the waves of life. They get back up on their board even as they anticipate the next wave. I recommend that you too, reclaim that *surfboard* and use it.

- Be courageous and interact with people. Don't worry if you think you are too sad or you have too red a nose from crying. No one really cares as they are often occupied with their own concerns.
- It is a gift that you are out there connecting. Both to you and to others.
- You will likely meet wonderful and caring people.
- You may experience your community as family.
- If you are lucky enough to have family, you may experience them as community.
- You may be surprised that you can be open to new interests, new types of recreation, creativity, situations, and people.

Life, abundant people, and love are really all around you and you can be buoyed by the waves.

You've got this!

In the next chapter about managing your well-being, you will receive useful tips in dealing with some of the more common challenges experienced by people who are grieving. These are based on my own experience and knowledge about health. Those who adopt healthy choices seem more resilient and better equipped to manage their grief and their future.

Your Well-being While Grieving

If we could give every individual the right amount of nourishment and exercise, not too little and not too much, we would have found the safest way to health.
HIPPOCRATES

PERHAPS YOUR LOVED ONE'S DEATH WAS CAUSED by an accident, sudden death, a short illness, or a long illness that took a turn. Whether you are forewarned of your loved one's health status and you anticipate their death or if the death is sudden, death brings sadness. The finality of death, even when it is anticipated, almost always brings a sense of shock.

There are many ways you can address your emotional and physical well-being following the death of your loved one. You may already have your own successful methods in place such as a daily yoga practice, prayer, or connection with your inner circle of close friends and family members. Or maybe you just hug your dog or cat.

As you begin to discover the new way to grieve that I describe in this book, it is important that you take care of your well-being at the same time. In this chapter I outline largely personal and anecdotal actions which I found to be helpful as certain issues seem to affect people who are grieving. I hope you try out any ideas that make sense for you. You can keep adding and use this list when you are ready to make a change or an addition.

Most important for your overall well-being is to be gentle with yourself and to be flexible. It may be important to set up your life to get support during the waves of grief. Cut yourself some slack. Be kind and patient with yourself.

Physical well-being

Your appetite may be affected. Your stomach might be upset. You may not be hungry, or you may eat more. Just go with it. If you are lucky to have people around, ask one person to be on the lookout for your nutrition and to bring you healthy food. Have people shop for you if possible.

Accept that your sleep is likely to be irregular. You may have difficulty getting to sleep or staying asleep, and you may awake early. You may experience early morning crying spells. This is all normal. Just knowing this might help you navigate. Having overnight company is great, but not as a guest who needs to be entertained. Any company who comes over, day or night, is not a guest per se, but someone who is there to comfort you. Please keep that in mind and allow them to do that. You are not in a host(ess) role now.

If you do not have to take pills for sleep, that is best. If you awake early, so be it. To help with maintaining a sleep cycle, when you do arise, go to the window and look out at the light of day, using this light to 'set' your circadian rhythm so that at sundown you begin to feel tired.

You may want to take a hot shower or bath an hour or so before bed. And it is best to not engage in any additional planning or stressful conversations especially at bedtime.

Some people like tart cherry juice concentrate an hour before bed, which provides natural melatonin, antioxidants, and a bit of sugar for a great combination of a blood sugar rise and fall for sleep. Downloading a light-dimming app like Flux to your computer or phone keeps your pineal gland from being stimulated and thus helps for deeper and more restorative sleep.

Visit your doctor for a baseline checkup if you can. He or she may know you well and offer some support and advice. Because of the stress, it is common to have some physical issue arise. If you have any pre-existing condition, it can 'kick up' during this stressful time of grief.

One friend shared that she had sudden bleeding and went for tests. Her diagnosis was kidney stones caused by not drinking enough water. Ironically, her late husband used to place a small pitcher of water in her home office daily, always kidding her that she did not drink enough water.

Emotional Well-being

Please be sure to exercise as you may have done prior to the death of your loved one and do whatever activity you feel up to doing. Releasing endorphins and maintaining your workout routine can be helpful to your state of mind and can also enhance your vitality.

You may hyperventilate or feel that you get upset very quickly. If so, you can place your hand on your abdomen and watch your stomach go up and down. You can pretend to blow out the candles on a birthday cake. Doing these things can slow your breathing, resolve your light-headedness, and even calm you.

In those first weeks and months I recommend you avoid any self-medicating substances, including alcohol. There will be time to imbibe if you like after grief ebbs, when you are feeling happier in your life. Drinking alcohol now can intensify your emotions, make you crave more alcohol (not good for your organs), upset your sleep quality, and render you ill-prepared to deal with your sadness.

Ask your doctor about taking vitamin D3. It is given according to your weight, health, and your current vitamin D level. D3 is a hormone and can help with your mood and has been known to prevent various diseases too.[3]

Taking a daily probiotic and having a balanced gut microbiome can be beneficial for your mindset too if your physician agrees. The stomach is sometimes called the 'second brain' due to the vagus nerve, which runs from your stomach right to your brain.[4] Optimized gut flora can also prevent illness and ward off inflammatory processes that you may be at risk for during the stress time of grief. If you are not functioning, not eating, not sleeping, inconsolable, or if you are experiencing signs of depression, hopelessness, or having thoughts of injuring yourself or others, *seek help from a competent professional immediately.*

I recall sharing that it was awful being on my own and not having Tom asking what I was planning for my day each morning. I told Laughlin Artz[5] I was concerned that I had no one to know what I was up to daily. Or worse, what if something happened to me? He suggested I

---

[3] Kranjac, P (2015, April 15). *The ABCs of Vitamin D with Dr. Michael Holick* [Video]. YouTube. https://youtu.be/LMos4WBxJoY

[4] Underwood, Emily. "Your Gut Is Directly Connected to Your Brain, by a Newly Discovered Neuron Circuit." *Science*, September 26, 2018. https://www.sciencemag.org/news/2018/09/your-gut-directly-connected-your-brain-newly-discovered-neuron-circuit.

[5] Seminar Leader, Landmark Worldwide.

ask someone to check in with me every morning for the next weeks or months.

I never would have come up with this incredible idea myself and I wondered who I could even ask to do this. It seemed intruding to ask of someone. I finally asked my friend Keith if he would be willing. Of course, he said yes. These generous morning 'check-ins' from Keith gave me huge peace of mind. It did not matter if he and his wife were traveling or local, he called me every day for six months. This seemingly small ritual made an enormous difference in my life. It is helpful if your friend is a good listener and allows you to cry if you need to. Your friend can support you in planning your day and taking new steps in your life. Support in the mornings and evenings or whenever you need it is so important.

You may have had an extreme change in lifestyle. You may now be living alone or sleeping alone maybe for the first time in decades. This was the case for me. I worked from home during the day and I did not want to be home at night too.

So, I made plans to pursue artistic and cultural interests outside of my home during the early evening when I would have usually been with my husband. My neighbor Denise rearranged her family life to come over every evening when I returned home from cultural outings. When time permitted, we would share a pot of peppermint tea. I would slice up some Bartlett pears and we would hang out. She listened to the story of my day, my sadness, my adventures, my concerns, and my dreams for the future.

These evening visits were life-enhancing touchpoints that I came to count on for months. While I could not have my husband, having a very kind, compassionate, and supportive neighbor over to my house consistently during those first few months was extraordinarily helpful for my well-being. You may have a solid support system already in place. If not, you can set up support – even if it does not seem like you can.

Look at what daily touchpoints you need and see what you can put in place. Even though this may seem a big 'ask' of another, friend and relative check-ins can be life preserving right now so be bold and ask! People can be big-hearted and helpful and many understand your situation and would be delighted to support you.

You can also set up hobbies at home and invite people to join you. I organized a small weekly art group for a handful of friends and neighbors. We met for an hour every week and made holiday cards. By doing so I had wonderful companions weekly to connect with and share our mutual interests right in my home. I was able to utilize the apartment space, especially my husband's den, in a new way and create new memories.

It was interesting for me to see that people who stepped up to be supportive of me had known grief at earlier stages of their lives. People who are there for you now may not be the people you expected to be there for you and may have even been strangers in your life before this. This can feel like a miracle and might turn into a profound bond lifelong.

Having a pet is another thing you can do for yourself. Pets love to be loved. I loved having my sweet Shih Tzu, Sandi. She was a wonderful source of added comfort and calm for me. She knew my cries and would come over to me when I was sad. Holding and hugging your pet produces oxytocin, "the love hormone," which is a wonderful antidote to cortisol, the stress hormone prevalent during grief.[6]

---

6   Oxytocin can also be produced from hugs by people you love, from making love, and from nursing a baby.

New Way to Grieve

I recommend meditation, especially Transcendental Meditation, which I do. You can do T-M anywhere. It has been scientifically proven to benefit and enhance your brain, body, and overall wellness. Though it is a time investment of 20 minutes twice daily, and costs money to learn, T-M has been studied and peer-reviewed by hundreds of health professionals and with data that backs up its promise for overall health benefits.[7]

You can be trained in other types of meditation, or even download meditation apps. One I recommend is called Calm. The app checks in with you at intervals, gauges your mood, and provides guided meditations to suit. You need to carve out the time to do this and the app has a monthly fee.

You might try a bereavement group especially if it deals with considering your future in addition to mourning the past. Look for a group that is hopeful and engages you in nudging you toward what is next. Choose one where you can connect with others and share. Caution: it is best to not use a bereavement group for a pity party. You may want to feel sorry for yourself, but that is a one-way ticket to additional misery.

While you might remind yourself that this is normal sadness and you may not need to *'fix it,'* treatment from competent grief-trained professionals helps many people. Perhaps it can help you too. Find a therapist you can trust. And one who actively supports you in creating a bit of joy for yourself or finding things that can enrich you or help you move forward in your life.

This is probably not the time to watch violent or scary movies or listen to upsetting things on the news. Avoid people who are negative about life. These can be triggers, so why put yourself through this? You may

---

7   Rosenthal, Norman E. *Transcendence: Healing and Transformation Through Transcendental Meditation.* TarcherPerigee; Illustrated edition (2012).

have difficulty focusing anyway.

You may want to clear out areas in your house that are filled with painful memories. Do this with others helping you if possible. Clearing out things by yourself can bring on extreme stress. Do this when you are ready. My friend Lydia terms this organizing a "cleaning posse," a supportive team of people who genuinely care about you and who are not affected by the space you are downsizing. I advise doing this process with relatives if there are no interpersonal issues coming to the foreground during this grieving time.

If you are living with others, especially your children, I recommend writing daily in a gratitude journal for those who live with you. Show it to them periodically. Or leave it where they can read it. Invite them to write in the journal similarly about what they appreciate. While others are reading about your gratitude, they will also be apt to acknowledge the difference you make to them too. They may be more comfortable writing than saying this to your face and the relationship can be enhanced. In general, everyone wants to hear what you mean to them; this is a great 'under the radar' but effective way to communicate especially when you are sad from grief.

If you are spiritual or religious, seek this type of support out for sure. You can attend spiritual classes or religious observances in person or on Zoom.

Finally, trust that you will be okay. Pull for yourself. If you do, likely it will not take long for you to be truly okay. I have been through this personally.

Here is a recap of some options to enhance and protect your physical and emotional well-being:

- Have someone check in with you every morning for one to six months. It can be brief, something to look forward to and provides daily connection and structure.
- Set up hobbies at home and invite others; create new memories and connections in your living space.
- Enjoy a pet.
- Be your own best friend. Be easy on yourself for what you can and cannot do. Be flexible with changes in how you eat and how you sleep.
- Get a baseline checkup with your doctor.
- Exercise daily if that is your usual practice.
- Do not drink or medicate unless necessary. And no scary movies for you right now.
- Meditate.
- Gather a "cleaning posse" rather than downsizing alone.
- Write in a gratitude journal daily.
- Attend spiritual or religious observances if that is your practice.
- Trust that you will be okay. Know that sadness is normal. Allow for it.
- If you experience thoughts of hurting yourself or anyone else, seek immediate help.

Tell yourself you can do this and take action!

In the next chapter I will define the concept of grief and sadness in contrast to thoughts and worries.

You may find this freeing!

What Is Grief?

Life imposes things on you that you can't control, but you still have the choice of how you're going to live through this.
CELINE DION

CULTURALLY, WE DO NOT USE THE WORD GRIEF accurately, and in fact, we have no shared definition. Concepts such as fear, worry, and even sleeplessness get rolled into the description. So how can we define grief?

One wellness website defines grief:

> ...a natural response to loss...the emotional suffering you feel when something or someone you love is taken away. Often, the pain of loss can feel overwhelming. You may experience all kinds of emotions, from shock or anger to disbelief, guilt, and profound sadness.

While I am not criticizing this website, its definition of grief is a perfect demonstration of how we sometimes explain our loved ones' death to ourselves. While perhaps it is not meant to, this definition perpetuates the likelihood of becoming trapped in our grief.

Within the words "suffering, love taken away, feeling overwhelmed, difficult and unexpected emotions, disbelief, guilt" is a potential trap where we may become stuck with more than just sadness. We do not even realize that these words can provide a hopeless way of coloring life and that then can affect our decisions about our future.

The word grief comes from the Latin word *gravare*, which means "to make heavy." *Gravare* itself comes from the Latin word *gravis*, which means "weighty." We can think of grief as *a heavy sadness*.

It is my opinion that pure grief is sadness. Grief is not all the tales that may get woven up in it. When someone we are close to dies, we usually have intense emotions, a rush of thoughts, regrets perhaps, and we have worries about how life may change. At times there is shock and anger.

Here is what grief is not: it is not that someone you love "was taken away." Likely, no one came and did that. In the reality that I call "pure grief," your loved one died.

Grief is not feeling overwhelmed. Merriam-Webster defines overwhelmed in the context of grief as "overcome in thought or feeling." Overcome is defined as "overpowered." More often, it is outside forces that can overpower someone. Thoughts and feelings are internal, and people have a choice about how to react to them. However, we do sometimes act like thoughts and feelings can overpower us.

If you choose to, you can tell yourself you are overwhelmed and overpowered. This is an example of telling yourself a *tale*. Then, you may take actions in accordance with feeling overwhelmed such as lying in bed all day or excessively eating or drinking with the intention of calming yourself or feeling something other than purely sad.

Curious about the words we tell ourselves, I read up on animal grief — where we only witness their behavior. In the first moments, there seems an awareness that their fellow animal has changed. The other animal is altered, not responsive, and their scent changes. Some survival responses

What is Grief?

to these changes seem protective in nature and involve cleaning debris[8] from the corpse, avoiding the site where the death occurred, and/or staying beside the animal that died.[9] Some responses seem related to survival such as sensing out the threat that killed their fellow animal, possibly to avoid it themselves. Within many animal species, the death of a family or pack member relates to a decrease in eating patterns, atypical squealing/wailing vocalizations, and lowered heads and tails.[10] Some of the scientific literature still couches animal behaviors with anthropomorphic labels like "depressed," making it difficult to really measure sadness in animals.

I recall burying my husband with my Shih Tzu in my arms. First she barked at the casket. Then she put her paw on it and made wailing-type noises which I had not heard from her before. It seemed she sensed or smelled Tom. She seemed to experience sadness. For weeks afterward, she went around the house looking for Tom and sniffing his things. She expanded her search all around in our neighborhood doing the same. Recently, she locked her eyes on a male neighbor as he carried a briefcase down into our former neighborhood garage. He resembled my husband in stature and it seemed my dog was attentive to that, even years after she had last seen Tom.

Then just two months ago, my pup ran over to me and barked when she heard me using Tom's nail clippers, apparently recognizing the sound associated with him.

Personally, I could identify early on that my dog was grieving and sad. She followed me around more, searched and sniffed Tom's things more, did not eat her dinner much for a time, and vocalized more.

---

8   Pierce, Jessica. "Do Animals Experience Grief?" *Smithsonian.com*, Smithsonian Institution, 24 Aug. 2018, www.smithsonianmag.com/science-nature/do-animals-experience-grief-180970124/.
9   van Leeuwen, E., Cronin, K. & Haun, D. Tool use for corpse cleaning in chimpanzees. *Sci Rep* 7, 44091 (2017). https://doi.org/10.1038/srep44091
10 Bekoff, Marc. "Grief in Animals: It's Arrogant to Think We're the Only Animals Who Mourn." *Psychology Today*, Sussex Publishers, 29 Oct. 2009, Landmark Worldwide Personal Performance Coaching

What goes wrong with sadness sometimes is that we attach other descriptive words and phrases to describe our sadness and those words disturb us. Then our behavior follows. Most of us do not consider what our words do to affect our feelings, which then impact our actions. We are not aware that we add what I call 'secondary thoughts and worries' to our sadness.

Words and phrases describing 'worries' about our future, ideas that 'we failed,' that we should feel 'shame and/or blame,' we experience 'fear' of being alone, we tell ourselves 'we cannot go on,' we say, 'we do not belong here anymore' or 'the world doesn't understand.' These things we also name 'grief.' Yet, mostly in my opinion, these thoughts *are not* grief. They are thoughts and concerns about what might arise. We all have them. We get so caught up in our thoughts about what might happen that the entire cauldron of emotions other than sadness can take over and may seem impossible to distinguish from our pure sadness.

We cannot control our thoughts. If we want to live with the idea that life is for the living, that we can look forward to a future for ourselves, and we can really choose being alive even if our loved one is not, we need to separate our thoughts about how things seem to be, or how things could turn out, from our pure sadness.

Though this may sound like it could take years to accomplish, the good news is that it does not need to.

Four months seems to be a turning point for many, when the reality hits. And indeed, four months after my husband died and after I sorted out the logistics and took care of so many details, I experienced sudden, enormous sadness and huge fear. The permanence of Tom's absence suddenly *leveled* me. He was never coming home. I was never going to have him in my life again. I would never see him again. I called Armand DiCarlo, someone I had known and trusted over many decades.[11]

---

[11] Landmark Worldwide Personal Performance Coaching.

What is Grief?

I told him, "Armand, I have handled the shock and the aftermath...but my life is over, I have no Tom, no husband!"

He remarkably helped me in one phone call to disentangle my sadness from my thoughts about Tom's death.

He said, "Paulette, look in the mirror. You are alive! It's true that you can create something new, it is not true that your life is over!" And with that, we began to look at what could happen in my future.

My gratitude for Armand's precious support has enabled me to be where I am today: happy, healthy, strong, and actively engaged in creating my life and future. And as such I am committed to sharing this journey and what I have learned that works.

I learned that:

- Grief is sadness. It can be extreme sadness.
- Grief is not thoughts about how things seem or worries about what might arise.
- Attaching thoughts and worries to sadness can disturb us.
- We can get stuck with worries and talk about them or complain to others and not take action to make things better for ourselves.

You are off to a wonderful start!

In the next chapter, we will drill down on what I call 'secondary thoughts' — thoughts we add to our sadness. By catching yourself hearing these secondary thoughts and worries, you may begin to gain some power over them.

This is an important chapter. Ready? Let's go!

Thoughts and Worries

If you could read my mind, love
What a tale my thoughts could tell
Just like an old-time movie
About a ghost from a wishing well
In a castle dark or a fortress strong
With chains upon my feet
You know that ghost is me
And I will never be set free
As long as I'm a ghost, you can see.
GORDON LIGHTFOOT
'If You Could Read My Mind'

GRIEF IS SADNESS. When someone we love dies, grief is deep sorrow brought about by their death. That is it.

Though it may be uncomfortable, *experiencing grief is a natural gift to ourselves and to the memory of our loved one*. The process of grief provides the work for us to do to be at peace with what happened and to honor our loved one, which may then open doors for what might be possible in the future.

While there is nothing you can do to change your circumstances, there are things you can do to mitigate the thoughts and feelings of despair, hopelessness, fear and panic that can amplify and prolong your sadness. These 'secondary thoughts and worries' can become your *booby traps*. There is a marked difference between the feeling of pure sadness and our disturbing, if not plaguing, secondary thoughts and worries about the future — the ones that can leave us feeling vulnerable, weak, and stuck.

First, let us examine closely what I mean by a thought. A thought is an idea or opinion occurring suddenly in the mind. It is likely that you will have many thoughts about the fact that your loved one died. Human beings can conjure up many thoughts about the same thing. Even conflicting thoughts. We like the cold weather. Then the temperature drops, and we hate the cold weather. Or we love this about her and then we say we hate this about her. Thoughts are always occurring, and some are ever-changing.

Worries are a state of anxiety and uncertainty over actual or potential problems. The outcome has not yet occurred and nonetheless, we can become focused on the worry instead of using it as a signal to take an action.

To demonstrate this more clearly, I have assembled a list of actual thoughts and worries that people grieving have shared. You may be able to identify some of these as ones you have heard or had yourself.

As you read these, see if you can recognize that these are *thoughts* and not *pure sadness*.

Within each statement or question below can you hear concerns and thoughts about the past and apprehensions about the future?

- I do not know what to do.
- My life is over.
- What is the point of living without him/her?
- I will never find love again.
- Who would want a widow with three young kids anyway?
- How can I ever love anyone else?
- She was my everything. She was my life.
- My ability to love died with them.
- I do not want to go on living without him/her.
- I lost my heart.
- How will I manage?
- A piece of me died with them.
- She was my soulmate.
- My heart is broken. There is a hole in my heart.
- This is breaking me.
- Someone tore me down this week.
- I loved them too much.
- I am waiting. I do not know for what.
- No one really understands me.
- If only they had/had not done, they would be alive.
- If only I had/had not done, they would be alive.
- I just cannot go on.
- Being a widow(er) is very hard.
- Grief never ends. I am forced to go through grief.
- I am struggling to find my way.
- I am a rockstar widow. People point at me in gatherings rather than include me.
- It is a brave new world.
- The space is too big to live in myself and I am frightened.
- I have so much to get rid of.
- I do not want to get rid of anything.
- People are mean and they rub salt on the wound.
- I want to see someone else get over what I must deal with.

Thoughts and Worries

- I feel like I am drowning all alone in this big world.
- Do not let anyone steal your joy.

Can you begin to realize some of your own concerns, your own thoughts?

It is my experience that when we dwell in thoughts and concerns, we prevent ourselves from releasing our sadness and that is where we may remain trapped, feeling vulnerable or powerless.

Is there really 'joy to steal'? How would one even do that? Break into your home and pull out the joy? This is illogical. Is there someone tearing you down and turning your life upside down? Is there struggle or a hole in your heart? Are you really drowning? All alone? I thought I was all alone too and then I went outside. There are tons of people around!

The good news of course is that thoughts and worries can be identified and addressed separately from your grief. I did not want to be stopped by nor stuck in my thoughts. This required doing 'word surgery' on myself — separating my sadness from my thoughts and worries. I noticed that I came to hear my same thoughts and worries every day and I wanted to speak them to anyone who would listen. I had to put the brakes on myself knowing that my words could create what I was concerned might happen. So, I began saying things like, "I am closing on my apartment in two months." Rather than my actual thought which was, "Who knows when I will close?! I am terrified of the interest and principal that is now due in a real estate market that is declining."

Writing these down and seeing them for what they are may allow your grief to surface. It is important to allow for and to express your sadness.

Try this:

Draw three columns. In the first column, make a list of words that you use to describe your sadness. In the second column, see if you can write down your thought that flows with the type of sadness you are experiencing. In the third column, write the worry that follows that thought. Keep listing these. Your three columns will contain these headings:

SADNESS	THOUGHT	WORRY
Deep sadness	No one will ever love me again	I will be alone forever

Go to the mirror or get with a friend and read the columns out loud. Notice that your sadness is grief and that the thoughts and worries are not.

You have now *separated* your thoughts and worries from your sadness. Keep noticing when the waves of sadness come up and if you are saying things to yourself that you think and worry about.

Practicing this is key to being able to grieve in a new way and not get stuck in your thoughts and fears.

Right now, the important work is to separate your thoughts and worries from your pure sadness.

Keep noticing if you have the same thoughts and fears over and over. Or do they change? Can you begin to identify a theme with which you concern yourself? Can you see that your thoughts and worries are unique to you?

Please do this exercise over the next several days in your journal as well. Continue to separate the sadness from the thoughts and worries you notice.

Thoughts and Worries

When we utter thoughts and worries to ourselves or others, we can get stuck believing them. Then we may find ourselves taking no action or taking a feeble action because we already have in mind that life is not going to turn out well for us. We let our words define the situation or ourselves, then react emotionally to the picture we painted.

Many people get immersed in their thoughts and concerns. They live life going through the motions, non-functional, hopeless, exhausted for decades or even a lifetime. It is my experience that people's spirits *die* not because of their sadness but because of the thoughts and worries they have about their circumstances which they believe to be real.

Key takeaways:

- Thoughts will undoubtedly intervene as they do for everyone. You may now see that you do not have to allow thoughts to sabotage you. By asking *"are those thoughts really true?"* and consistently identifying them when they surface and avoiding giving in to them, you may see you have power over them. Catch yourself!
- Be sad when you are sad. Realize you have a choice to just be sad instead of getting immersed in secondary thoughts and worries. If you find you are stuck, ask yourself what you gain by adding frightening and despairing thoughts to feelings of sadness and missing your loved one. This is the hard work of separating upsetting thoughts from sadness.
- Worries can be an alert that there is something you might want to do instead of feeling scared about something that hasn't happened yet (and may not ever happen). While we cannot prevent thoughts and worries from occurring, we do not have to believe them nor allow them to trap us into feeling hopeless, resigned, helpless, fearful, anxious, panicked or worried.

- Can you notice any thought patterns that recur which disturb, haunt, or derail you the most?
- Can you notice that someone in your exact same situation may not have any of the thoughts that you have? If you can also see this, you might get a glimpse of your point of view and begin to watch for it. This is *advanced* reflection and can be very freeing.

You have done some very keen work here!

Many times, during grief there are miscommunications and dashed hopes at a time when you may need connection the most. The next chapter is about hearing the 'music' from others and not just the 'words' so you can stay connected, because as you know, others have thoughts and worries too!

Staying Connected Regardless of Others' Thoughts

> *Keep smiling, keep shining*
> *Knowing you can always count on me, for sure*
> *That's what friends are for*
> *For good times and bad times*
> *I'll be on your side forever more*
> *That's what friends are for.*
> BURT BACHARACH & CAROL BAYER SAGER
> 'That's What Friends Are For'

OTHERS' WORDS AND DEEDS MATTER and we often wish that everyone would be on our side 'forever more' as the song says.

When my husband died suddenly, a friend said to me, "At least he is in a better place now." Aghast at first, I thought, "What? How can she say that? He was not ill. Further, how can he be in a better place if not with me? We were so happy together. Wouldn't he have wanted me in this *better place* with him?"

Then I realized that this friend did not understand the impact of her words and that she just did not know what else to say. I could hear that she was trying to be gracious and comfort me as her beliefs dictated. I realized then that we do not have to allow others' words or beliefs upset us.

I wished she had said something like this:

> I hear you are very sad. He was your soulmate over four decades. The future may seem very scary to you right now. I am here for you. I will call you every week. Tell me more about your feelings, your concerns, your worries. We will get through this together!

In this example, my grief would be acknowledged. My friend would have helped distinguish my thoughts from my sadness. Finally, and importantly, I would be reassured by her availability, support, and commitment to me. This is a huge gift to hear someone and be here for someone![12]

I have come to see that the most useful thing is for someone to listen to you without judging, without making suggestions, without feeling sorry for you and without interpreting anything from their own viewpoint. Having someone listen actively without attempting to say something simply because they want to comfort you is ideal.

People who care about you may just want to say *something*. They may not be aware of how their words come across to you, especially now when you are grieving. It is important that when others share their thoughts that you hear them as just thoughts. Try thinking of it this way, if someone says that by rubbing a rabbit's foot you will encounter a million dollars or that Santa Claus is really coming to town, it's preposterous. It can be easy to embrace that their thoughts and words are not necessarily things you need to believe as true.

---

[12] Grief Recovery Method

Staying Connected Regardless of Others' Thoughts

Keep in mind that while people may have good intentions, they may not understand. Most times they have not had your *exact* circumstances. This is important to note as I have witnessed many times that people who are grieving find themselves angry at people who don't seem to understand and who may say the wrong things in the wrong way or at the wrong time. What is worse is that this is a time when someone grieving may want to be closer to others and receive their support.

I erred in my late 20's attempting to provide comfort for an older mother who had miscarried, though had previously conceived one child. My caring and comforting words were not received as I meant them to be when I offered that she would most likely conceive again given she had done so before. *What suddenly made me the 'conception expert' instead of a compassionate friend?* I learned my lesson!

People who are grieving only want to be heard for their feelings and for what matters to them. They want to know that you care and the degree to which you can be supportive.

And as a listener, people want to be comforting and may indeed not have the right words. People have thoughts and you don't have to allow the thoughts to impact you.

Others' thoughts that I have heard and read:

Here's what I think you should do. Here's what you should not do. You are too sad, too alone, too depressed, too happy, too thin, too fat, too poor, too worried, too sedentary. You are leaning on your kids too much, going out too much, talking too much about your feelings, talking too much about your personal finances.

You are taking too long — it is six months already, haven't you moved on? You are not eating healthfully enough, not exercising enough, not spending time productively enough. You're too poor and unfortunate, too much to deal with.

Why don't you sell your home? Why would you move? You are spending your money too fast. You are a great catch. I can't imagine if this ever happened to me how I would handle it.

Your kids' thoughts:

You are doing it all wrong. You are being annoying. Why are you still being so sad? You are being too joyful. Why are you having a date so soon? Why are you interacting with me so much? Why do you leave me alone so much? You are not even concerned about my feelings. You should not be on Bumble or Tinder! Why are you depending on me to be your sounding board? You need therapy!

In the case of a spousal loss, your spouse's family's thoughts:

Why are you tossing out clothing and personal items? Why did you give away all her things? You probably did not love her enough; you could have done more to help her live. We never liked you anyway. You got the wrong doctor. You are selfish. Why did you get rid of all his photos in the house? We are not inheriting anything from you. We no longer must ask you to family gatherings now that s/he is gone. You are his second wife, and we will make sure you don't collect anything in the will as we are his children. We don't think you should be dating and if you are, keep it to yourself!

Staying Connected Regardless of Others' Thoughts

Your married friends' thoughts:

Certainly, we will be there for you...at least now. But then you will be a single man, a third wheel to us and our friends. You will be dating, and you are a bachelor, and it won't be appropriate to have you join us, it will make us uncomfortable. You have other friends by now I am sure. We can invite you over when we have other friends visit who lost their spouses. You are too sad to be around. We miss your spouse too.

When I got divorced people no longer included me, so I won't include you. You are no longer included in our inner circle because it is too hard to deal with you now. You are attractive, and you may be attracting my wife/husband, so I will not allow you as our friend.

There are hundreds if not thousands of thoughts that we could come up within an hour.

Multiply this by how much time and by how many people are in your life and you could experience yourself becoming a prisoner of your thoughts and the thoughts of others.

What to know:

- Allow people to listen to you. Understand that it is common to *not feel heard* during this time. People who have loved ones die often say, "No one understands me, how could they?" People do try to listen, and many have their own agenda and their own reactions. If they do not understand, just tell them again.
- Have compassion for *others* even though it is *you who are* grieving. People sometimes say their thoughts out loud. You don't have to

believe the thoughts. Just note that they are speaking to you and they seem to care no matter how awkward their words seem.
- Remember, it is the music rather than the words. That is to say, it is *that* they are saying something, not so much *what* they are saying.
- People may have difficulty finding the right things to say. The death of your loved one is upsetting for them as well. Give them space and don't react to what they say. They don't mean it to hurt you.

Great work in drilling down on the thoughts of others, not taking them as something to believe, and staying connected as much as possible. This is very important now!

In the next chapter we can begin to look at what you might wish for your future!

A 'Wish List' for Your Future

When you wish upon a star
Makes no difference who you are
Anything your heart desires
Will come to you.
NED WASHINGTON
'When You Wish Upon a Star'

IT IS NOW TIME TO TAKE A CHANCE AT CREATING. Let's peek at the things you may want in your life and the future you might fashion.

How to Create a 'Wish List' If You Are Sad

Focus on considering your *wishes* for today. This is a preliminary wish list. You can begin to look at anything you would like to have in your life. First, try doing it quickly.

Whatever comes to mind, write it down. This is not about getting it right. It's about getting it done.

Do you want to be living near your friends or children? Do you want a new pet? Is there a dream vacation that you imagine? You may want a romantic relationship. Write everything down, uncensored on a fresh piece of paper. Thoughts and opinions will intervene, you can count on that. Just write down what you *think you want* anyway. Take a chance to create something for the future.

Replace the worried thoughts and phrases, such as "I will never love again" or "My life is over" with what you might want in your future, such as "I want love in my life" or "I would love to have more friends to do things with!"

Thoughts are powerful and may create exactly the future you describe. Our thoughts can become our mantra, and if we speak them, they may become more real to yourself and to the others who hear them. Write your wish list and seal it in an envelope. Open it six months from now. You may be surprised to realize what you really want in your life and how much you could even consider for yourself within the first few months of grief. Later, we will look closer at what fits your life. For now, just write down anything that comes to mind.

Try this:

- Free associate. Just start writing.[13]
- Some things may come up that surprise you. That's okay. Just write it anyway. This is the time for you to create — just like painting on a new canvas.
- It doesn't have to be perfect. Allow yourself to dream a little bit. More dreaming will come later.
- Seal your letter and open it in six months.

---

13 Thomas Rabeyron and Claudie Massicotte. "Entropy, Free Energy, and Symbolization: Free Association at the Intersection of Psychoanalysis and Neuroscience", 17 Mar. 2020, 11:366, doi: 10.3389/fpsyg.2020.00366. eCollection 2020.

A 'Wish List' for Your Future

How exciting and powerful it is to see that you can create a preliminary wish list for your life, regardless if you are sad. Extremely well done!

Hang on for the next chapter about forgiving your loved one. More powerful work on grief is about to come and can provide peace of mind!

Anger First, Then Forgiving Your Loved One

*When a deep injury is done to us,
we never heal unless we forgive.*
NELSON MANDELA

IT MAY SEEM HARDLY APPROPRIATE OR EVEN WRONG to feel anger when your loved one dies. However, anger does surface, even at them. To move forward in your life, it is important to realize and express the anger you may have. It is very common to be angry with yourself, too.

Though you cannot speak in person, and this is a one-way communication, it is critical to adopt forgiveness to move forward.

- First, reflect on your anger at them when they were alive.
- Then consider your anger now due now due to their death.
- Finally, focus on the anger that surfaces as you envision your future without them.

Anger About the Past

You may be angry that your loved one died. This did not have to happen. Your life has not been fair. It is not fair that they died.

You may have anger that perhaps your loved one:

- Neglected their health or embraced the wrong health habits prior to their death.
- Ignored early warning signs and mismanaged their own well-being.
- Received the wrong medical advice from less than competent professionals.
- Incurred a disaster or preventable injury or took a calculated risk!

You may be angry about how your loved one handled their health as they were dying. Maybe they refused the medical team you took the time to gather, the experts you thought could have preserved their dignity and saved their life. You may be angry at the physical and emotional exhaustion you felt with your specific challenges in life.

You may have anger at how helpless you felt or how draining it was to be their frontline caregiver. Maybe you are angry at how their other caregivers handled things.

You may be angry at how your loved one succumbed to death. Perhaps you are angry that no one was sensitive to what you were going through while your loved one was dying. You may have anger about the huge medical expenses incurred and the impact on you and the family.

You may feel angry that your loved one used poor lifestyle judgment, failed to exercise, refused to see doctors when they weren't feeling well, refused to communicate with you or professionals the extent of their concerns or pain.

Maybe they were out of shape and they exercised in an obscure area of town where no ambulance could locate them in time for defibrillation to save them. That was my husband's situation. On one hand, at 67, he was acting in line with good health choices and exercising. On the other hand, he was taking a calculated risk. Out of shape, he died on a tennis court in an obscure area where an ambulance came too late.

I experienced fury and rage from this gigantic, tragic, preventable, sudden, and precious loss. I was angry at him, his tennis partner, the public park where they played, the ambulance, and the government for not having defibrillators on the courts.

I had been worried and irritated during the days prior because he was moody and snappish, and I did not know why. Then of course I felt guilt. I had to forgive him and myself and all that I had been angry about.

Perhaps you think your loved one ignored sound medical advice or did not take their test results seriously enough. Maybe they did not behave as you think you would have in their position, or you think they should have.

You might blame your loved one for how they behaved during various phases of their illness. You may feel anger at how they treated you or how you saw them act toward other loved ones. You might have anger about what they said to you during their illness. A phrase or sentiment may resound repeatedly in your thoughts. You may wonder what they meant by something they said.

A friend told me that her mother said something that she construed as mean and hurtful in her final days and she could not even utter it aloud to me. She replayed the phrase to herself and wondered why her mother would leave her with such an apparently painful sentiment. Mean words can render lasting damage unless they are expressed and then forgiven. Forgiving provides freedom and peace of mind.

Otherwise, you could be left stuck and punishing yourself with hurtful sentiments your loved one may have stated before they died.

You may experience anger about what your loved one did not communicate, such as not fully expressing their love and gratitude for you. Perhaps they did not tell you fully or often enough what they loved about you, what they felt about their life with you.

Perhaps they did not tell others, such as their own children, how much they loved them, and this falls on you to reassure the children.

Maybe you are angry that they did not have enough time for you, and they did not acknowledge that to you. Or that they were not the family member or friend you wanted them to be and they wanted to be for you.

There may be incidents that occurred when your loved one was alive that never got spoken about even though they made you angry. You never expressed this anger to them.

Anger About Your Situation Now

If you look, you may find yourself angry about many different things right now.

Most significantly you may be very angry that you are now alone, you miss them, and you are grieving. You may be angry at how much there is to do and to deal with. Angry that they did not make it. Anger about what you must go through now. You may be angry at taking care of the kids now as you are sad and in shock. And you may be angry about burial wishes and plans not in order.

You may be angry at how they managed their life, their accounts, and affairs. You may be angry that you must downsize and deal with legal and financial issues and how they relate to your life now given your state of grief. You may be angry that they did not plan for your future. It may be unthinkable that there were papers unsigned and vague.

Someone on Facebook posted that she was left with many things to deal with after her husband's sudden death. There was debt, no life insurance, and a multitude of papers not in order. His kids were not accounted for in any will. Her husband was in his 50's and did not anticipate or consider end of life decisions. Specific anger about each of these issues may be present for her as well as anger associated with the lack of forethought and effort her loved one provided about their end-of-life circumstances.

One widow that I knew had a husband who died of COVID-19. She was wife number two and his will had been written in an obscure way. Though she had been in his life 28 years, his six offspring fought to keep her out of gaining any spousal benefits. This was extremely sad and anger-provoking for this widow.

Were there exorbitant medical bills left for you? Is your loved one's will fair to you? Did they endow someone other than you or have a previous family that will inherit money, leaving you financially insecure? Is the legal aftermath a complete surprise? And can you get into all their accounts or are you in a password protected nightmare?

Maybe you are angry that now, during your grief and sadness, you must move out because you cannot afford the current financial responsibility on your own. Maybe you are not assured inheritance of the property, or you lost your medical coverage, or your children are not being protected. Perhaps your loved one left you to care for their own sick child or their own ailing parent who still lives with you.

A widower told me his wife was a hoarder. It took him several years to downsize all her things. He was angry that she left these responsibilities to him. He was angry at how very sad and stressful it was for him to go through all her personal items and papers which also represented their memories together, such as every movie ticket stub, etc. He had to spend much time on this memory-painful process.

Anger As You Consider the Future Without Your Loved One

You may have thoughts about what the future may hold for you without your loved one. And that they now will not be a part of your children's future. All of this may have been unthinkable before and now you are dealing with anger at the reality of a future without them.

A widower I recently met, married 45 years to his high school sweetheart, had just retired from his medical practice. He was planning to relocate with his wife and travel the world. Then she died.

You may likely feel angry about what could have been, angry about what you may have been planning but now will never happen. You may be missing that person to love, to receive love from, to have fun with, to create future dreams with, to turn to in times of need or for advice, and to share hugs and support. You are missing the person with whom you were building life and the person who understood you like no one else. All your dreams of your loved one being there in your future are now changed.

Express Your Anger in Three Letters

This next exercise involves you writing *three* different personal letters to your loved one as though they were alive. Your anger needs to be expressed in words. This way you have a chance that your anger does not preoccupy you. Though you may not want to or feel it is wrong to express anger for your loved one right now, it is very important to recognize and articulate the anger. Releasing your thoughts and feelings of anger in this manner, can help you move through your grief.

Notice all the things you think "should have been" or "could have gone" or "if only it was this or that way." Once you have one thought, you may notice a stream of additional thoughts. You can add to the letters as more thoughts surface. This exercise might feel awkward but can be a key component of moving forward in your life.

Try this:

Please take out your journal. Using three clean pages, begin three letters to your loved one. Create a heading line stating what the letter is about.

LETTER ONE:
I am angry with you for what happened in the past.

> Dear Jack,
> How could you have taken the train that derailed when you were supposed to drive to work that day!!! I'm mad at you for having been angry at me these past few months!
> And that is was always about work with you! I'm upset that you yelled at the kids instead of having more patience. I am angry with you for drinking so much and not having

enough time for me. I'm angry that we never got to go to Alaska. I'm upset that I have to take care of our dog all alone. I hate that I felt lonely around you so much when you were alive. I hate that you took your mother's side about the mortgage payments. Why did you never tell me how much you loved me? I had to hear it from others.

LETTER TWO:
I am angry with you about what is happening in my life now.

> Dear Jack,
> I cannot believe after 30 years of marriage that you died. I cannot stand being without you. I am numb. I cannot deal with anything right now. This is such a big house. I can't believe I have to sleep by myself. I miss you. I cry all the time. I have no idea what to do. I can't function. I'm not eating. I'm cold. I'm scared. I'm angry. And lonely. I'm furious at you! I can't believe that you died.

LETTER THREE:
I am angry with you about my future.

> Dear Jack,
> Go on without you!? How!? I can't imagine that we won't grow old together. I thought this would be forever with you. I can't support this house by myself. I'm going to have to move. It's unthinkable that I would be a widow at my age. How am I going to raise our children by myself? And your mother is living with us! What am I going to do about that? This is awful. I'm so worried. This isn't how things were supposed to turn out. I am so angry at you and terrified of a future without you!

Doing this will enable you to release your anger and see more clearly what might be there to forgive. Keep writing until issues you have not even thought much about are written down. Include the ones that may seem petty, such as, they were always late and more significant ones such as they did not carry their weight financially and the pressure was on you.

Now try forgiveness:

- Get tissues ready. You might cry.
- Say out loud each thing you are angry about or read it in the mirror.
- If you can forgive that item, say "I forgive you for that."
- The more items you can forgive, the more peace of mind you may be able to achieve for yourself.
- Forgiving can provide you with an enhanced freedom to dream!
- This process may bring up some other feelings such as more anger, sadness, guilt, etc. Express it all.
- It is okay to let go of anger. It just takes you saying that you forgive — without any qualifiers. "I forgive, but…" is not forgiving.

If you cannot forgive them right now:

- Come back to that item later.
- Try applying a percentage to it. *"I 75% forgive you!"* Then look to see what the 25% left represents. By doing it this way, you might even lighten up about what you are angry about. "Whoa! I forgave all but 2%!" If that is the case, what possible grudge are you holding onto and would it be worth your freedom to forgive the remaining percentage?
- Consider if they did this on purpose. If that is the case, can you apply more reasoning and compassion? If not, can you be gracious and let it go and actively forgive knowing your compensation can be increased peace of mind for yourself?

Recently at a Zoom funeral, a daughter whose mother was an upstanding member of the community spoke in an angry, inappropriate way about her mother, saying that she was "complicated" along with other critiques. My concern was for the daughter who may be likely to have thoughts throughout her life about her mother with no love, forgiveness, or compassion.

If the daughter could write such a letter, perhaps she could gain some freedom and peace of mind regarding her mother and her mother's death. Perhaps then she could simply experience pure sadness. It was evident to me that the daughter was stuck in her past view of things with anger that was unexpressed, and she was trapped emotionally.

Anger can upset our peace of mind, block our creativity, and our ability to consider what is important to us. It can block our ability to feel love. Our anger can affect our health and long-term quality of life. Hence the expression, "She makes me sick!"

Express yourself in writing to your loved one with dementia.

There may have been limited time and ability to say what you wanted to say so that they could have heard you. If your loved one had dementia, you slowly said "goodbye" perhaps, but maybe you did not really communicate all you wanted to say to them.

You may be left holding onto the unexpressed love and gratitude that you have for them. Or any feelings for that matter.

Write all this down.

What of the death of a child?

As parents, our job is to love, protect, and raise our children to grow up and take complete care of themselves lifelong. If they die, we may naturally experience failure.

Twelve parents I know had their children die. There is complete anguish and sadness and much anger, blame, and shame that goes with this. At times, illness or even death of a parent can be the result or breakup of the marriage. I have seen it all.

There is work to do to forgive regarding your offspring who died. And forgiveness of yourself as a parent.

A distant cousin's troubled daughter died. My cousin called me, speechless, inaudibly whispering about her daughter's death and that she herself had laryngitis and now a vocal cord problem. By the end of the phone call of sharing about her daughter, the impact of this unexpected death, and what she herself regretted and forgave, suddenly my cousin's voice became her strong, audible voice again. She had now 'voiced' her thoughts and separated them out from the pure grief she had.

Regardless of who has died in your life, it is usually the same thing: forgive them, forgive yourself, express it all and move forward. We will speak about forgiving yourself in the next chapter.

What of a sudden tragic situation or unexpected accident?

There is not time to say all you have to express. There is not only loss. There are many more issues at play which may require forgiveness of yourself. At times, sudden grief is silenced. The blame felt by the survivor and shame attached to a suicide, for example, can sometimes invalidate a person's ability to further express themselves. Grieving can be stilted and so can the griever's quality of life for their future. Thoughts of blame and shame can indeed paralyze survivors of suicided loved ones or if loved ones exchanged cross words before one of them died. There is work to do to express anger and forgiveness.

I know a woman whose brother committed suicide. After his death, she moved far away, devoted her life to studying non-violent communication, engaged in many practices of healing and meditation. She is still consumed by her secondary thoughts and has not forgiven her brother or herself. Even though you may do things like move physically and change your focus, you may still be stuck unless you do the exercises and the work to feel pure grief and forgiveness so that you can move on emotionally.

Expressing yourself completely by way of writing these three letters is very important work for you now.

These exercises may feel upsetting, unnatural, and maybe even superfluous. I have found the exercises effective even though I had some of these same thoughts and opinions. Do them even if they feel uncomfortable or too time consuming. Once you do, you might be able to begin to formulate what you want in your life.

I am confident that you can do this.

Try this:

- Write your loved one three letters about your anger: one to them about past anger, one about present anger and one about anger you have about your future.
- Include every detail of what they did or did not do. Every detail of what they said or did not say and anything else that made or makes you feel angry.

- Realize that this is a healthy exercise to do. It does not mean you will stay angry at your loved one forever, or that that is the only feeling you have about them. Here we are focusing on anger.
- Read the letters out loud, preferably in the mirror.
- Try forgiving your loved one for each angry thing you wrote about, one by one. Say it like this, "I am angry that you did X and I forgive you for it."
- If you are not willing to forgive something now, that is fine. You can try again later.
- The more you can forgive, the more peace of mind, love and freedom you can experience.
- The more freedom you can experience, the more ability you may have to create something new.

You can do this! This is powerful! You are powerful!

When you forgive yourself, as we will cover in the following chapter, you may be more readily able to act upon the things you want to pursue in your life. Though this may sound strange, forgiving yourself can open you up to realizing what you deserve and give you the *oomph* to achieve what you want.

This next chapter is very compelling and effective for your future results. Just watch!

Anger, Then Forgiving Yourself

Sittin' in the mornin' sun
I'll be sittin' when the evenin' come
Watching the ships roll in
And then I watch 'em roll away again
I'm just sittin' on the dock of the bay
Wasting time.

OTIS REDDING, STEVE CROPPER
'(Sittin' On) The Dock of the Bay'

IT IS WHEN YOU FORGIVE YOURSELF that you can see that you deserve a future. You may then see you deserve to take actions to make that future great.

I hope you have done the work and have forgiven your loved one. Now it is time for the work to forgive yourself.

"What does it mean to forgive myself? I did not cause my loved one to die!", you might think. And yet many of us have thoughts that we could have done better, we could have done it differently, we could have done more of this and less of that. There were actions that you took. What is likely true is that you did your best with what you knew to do at the time. However, maybe some of the things you did and/or said do not sit perfectly right with you now.

Writing a letter to yourself is very effective for this exercise. Using your journal, write down everything that you are angry at yourself for.

- Write down what you did not do for your loved one that you regret not having done.
- Write what you did for your loved one that you regret, which it turned out, was not helpful to them.
- Write what you regret not saying, perhaps including acknowledging love and gratitude for your loved one.
- Write what you said that you regret. That which may not have been received well, such as complaints or anger.
- Go back through these sections and forgive yourself for each thing in your journal.

For example, the letter can begin with what you regret not having done:

> Dear Paulette:
> I am angry at myself that I did not do enough interacting with the doctors, that I did not insist enough on preventative care such as diet and exercise for you. I am angry at myself that when you did not listen to me, I was not able to influence you to adopt healthy lifestyle practices. I regret that I did and said nothing when you ate the entire two pies you received by mail. I am angry at myself that I did not pierce through your angry mood those last few weeks and get you to the doctor.

Whatever remorse, regret, or anger you have towards yourself for what you did or said or how you acted toward your loved one or did not act towards them, should be described fully in this letter.

Perhaps you think you added to your loved one's stress. That you did not contribute to their peace of mind. Maybe you feel you did not visit them enough where they were being cared for or could not be there due to outside circumstances. Perhaps you did not take their complaining seriously enough early on or that you did not respond swiftly enough or help them get to the best expert in the field. If you are a physician or a medical professional, you may be thinking that even though you were not their doctor, you should have and could have known or done more.

How about something inadvertent that you blame yourself for? One of my friends was dealing recently with a serious concussion and phoned me. "My wife has not slept in days. She knows that if she had pulled up the emergency brake in our new car in time, that when I opened the car door, the car would not have rolled down the hill, I would not have been thrown back nor hit my head nor incurred a major concussion."

To that I replied, "I am going to ask you a question to ask your wife. Did she really mean to not pull up the emergency brake?" The answer to the question is of course, obvious. To that he replied, "Perfect! I will let her hear it this way."

The message here is that while we do not mean to cause harm, we believe at times that we did harm. It is important to express that if it is the case and forgive, so that we do not blame ourselves further. In some cases, we do harm unknowingly by accident. Sometimes too, we say things we regret.

Maybe you think you were impatient, condescending, or intolerant at times. Maybe you believe that you reacted disdainfully or distantly toward your loved one while they were ill and or dying. Perhaps you were frightened of losing them such that you became distant to protect yourself.

Maybe their dementia had you rationalize that it was okay to disengage and withhold your love and not regularly visit them because you were convinced that they would not even notice. Identify even the smallest things you skipped doing such as not bringing them that protein shake when you knew it might help fortify them or not buying flowers to take to the hospital to express your love and brighten their day. You may feel you cut corners in demonstrating your love and caring. Note all of this in your journal and forgive yourself.

What if you corrected them or embarrassed them in front of someone else or made them feel sad, uncomfortable, and confused? Did you dredge up the past and get angry when you did not mean to?

Did you neglect to tell them about the gratitude and love you had for them, how wonderful they were to you, what they meant to you, how you felt about them? Maybe they loaned you money to launch your now-successful business, or they nudged you into taking piano lessons because they noticed you had talent.

What if your loved one died suddenly after you spoke harshly to each other? Often in undetected illness (*dis-ease*), irritability is present, and it seems difficult to communicate anything positive to the ill person. Forgive yourself any last interactions as well.

Maybe during their life, you did not take the time off to have that dream vacation with them, hear about their proudest moment one last time, or do that class they wanted you to do with them.

Write all your regrets down. This is not about blaming yourself. It is about seeing your thoughts and having the opportunity to forgive yourself for each regret if you have any. We may have thoughts that we did something terrible or simply that we could have done better. Sometimes these thoughts haunt us for days, weeks, months, or even years. Sometimes these thoughts paralyze us.

You might also like to write down how possibly relieving it is for you to express these facts to yourself – if it is.

Important to note that it does not matter if you think your loved one realized any difficult last interactions. This is about telling the truth to yourself.

This letter-writing exercise is the heavy lifting!

It is my experience that though it may be challenging to put words to these thoughts, this is this difficult work that needs to be done to feel free, at peace, and to grant yourself permission to dream and move forward.

Do your best to forgive each thing that you did or did not do and each thing that you did not say or did say. This is a critical piece of this exercise. What I discovered is that when we forgive ourselves, we can see that we deserve a future. We may then more clearly see the actions necessary to make that future great.

Read the letter line by line in the mirror preferably. See if you can forgive yourself for each item.

Notice if you cannot forgive something. Take a fresh look at that item later. See what percentage of that item you can forgive yourself for.

This exercise can be sad to do. We are human beings, and we are not perfect. There is an impact we have had on others and the world based on what we did or did not do. At the same time, this exercise can give you relief. It is valuable, courageous, big-hearted work which can move you forward in your life.

Forgiving yourself gives you the ability to make things happen. You may be amazed that the more you forgive yourself, the more you can feel like you *deserve* to take actions toward your dreams.

Well and honorably done!

In the next chapter we will discuss finding the things that fit your life now. You've got this.

Freedom to Dream to See What Fits You Now

City of Stars are you shining just for me?
City of Stars, there's so much that I cannot see. Who knows?
Is this the start of something wonderful and new?
BENJ PASEK AND JUSTIN PAUL
'City of Stars'

WHEN I WROTE MY ORIGINAL WISH LIST LETTER I had expressed that I wanted more friendships and many more people in my life, including a romantic relationship. I wanted to try doing things with others related to the arts and exploring things I had never done before. It was there on paper in my own words. Writing this letter, I had 'tried on' what I wanted in my life.

The first thing became clear to me — I did not want to be at home by myself in the evenings in a city apartment in which I had worked all day. "No one is going to ring my doorbell!" I thought. I needed to go out and discover life on my own.

I decided to not be home after my workday ended! And to explore a new venue every evening even if it only *mildly* interested me. In fact, I didn't even know what specifically interested me then anyway.

The word 'challenging' does not begin to describe the anguish I experienced daily as dusk approached. Further, due to so many previous deaths among family members and people in my life who divorced or moved away, I keenly knew I needed to build new friendships near where I lived.

All of this seemed rather *impossible* to me and way too big a challenge, especially around weekends and holidays. It was uncomfortable to leave my house most of the time. I was sad and embarrassed to show up in places where I did not know anyone, especially where there were couples. I did not want to be viewed as single and alone. And mostly I did not want anyone to feel sorry for me.

Freedom to Dream

I decided to keep myself focused on what interested me, on what was important to me, and on what could engage me. Happiness was not my concern. Engagement in things of interest was.

I gave myself permission to pursue a wide variety of venues regardless of whether it matched my old identity as *Paulette, partner for 43½ years to my husband*. After a while, I found myself able to envision a canvas to explore the world as wide and blank and many new interests and surprises appeared.

I took myself to dance venues and performances, art venues, galleries and museums, music events and concerts of all types and sizes from intimate rock and pop shows to large scale jazz and oldies performances. I went to lectures, art, and architecture tours. I visited Archtober, a great and diverse venue in October in New York. I went on historical tours, attended openings and performances in theatre, opera and ballet, and I visited a vast array of places of worship. It was all there for discovery. I was grateful to be in a rich city to locate anything I could imagine. Eventually I was courageously able to venture to a handful of neighborhood restaurants on my own.

I attended every event I was invited to and met up with any friend or acquaintance who asked me. I was unwilling to spend any evening home alone, even if it meant taking the subway to a new neighborhood and walking about on my own or being out when the weather was inclement.

On one such walk I heard jazz music playing from an open windowed bar on the second floor. I went inside. There I got to reconnect with Gene Bertoncini, the great American Jazz guitarist I had met 25 years prior. Quite unexpectedly, while mingling with others during the break, I was introduced to a physician neighbor of my husband's former boss at Columbia Presbyterian. This was an extraordinary experience that held many coincidences.

It may seem like I was easily able to go out and live life after my husband's death. It was quite the contrary. I could have readily let my thoughts keep me home alone and feeling sorry for myself. I pushed myself out the door nightly, just because I said I would do that. Because as I mentioned earlier, *no one was ringing my doorbell.*

To motivate myself particularly on holidays and special days, I would play the '*100 Years Game*' shared with me by my friend Ken. Subtracting my age from 100 I would tell myself, *"That leaves possibly 37 more New Year's Eves to enjoy, so get out and do it!"* This was both a good reality check and a way of getting myself out the door — life is finite and who even knows whether we have 100 years. This trick showed me I had a choice of how I want to live every day and every holiday too. You have a choice as well.

Two years after my husband died and after I completed all the logistical work from the aftermath of his death, I began to visit, explore, and dream about where I wanted to live. I considered potential career changes and enhancements and expansion of my relationships and personal growth.

Looking at your living situation, relationships, interests, career, personal growth, etc., take a page for each in your journal and spend a few minutes to consider what you want and what you can dream of for yourself. Try not to censor yourself thinking it is not possible. Just write down what you picture regardless of those thoughts.

Participating and sharing with others can be the gift you give yourself.

I discovered throughout my efforts to *try on what fit me now* that I did not need to hide my sadness or pretend I was not grieving. You do not need to put on a happy face just to be welcomed by people. If you have the courage to move outside your door despite your thoughts and sadness, you can more fully be living life, even if you do not have a plan. It takes willingness, courage, and heart.

Going out and exploring on my own is how I learned I could be myself with people even in my sadness and share my thoughts, feelings, and circumstances. I realized from people's reactions and expressions that it was not typical to encounter a 63-year-old widow, suddenly alone after a long happy marriage, out and about and moving forward in life. I saw that sharing with others was inspiring to people. For some, it prompted their own sharing about things that were sad or traumatic in their lives. I soon discovered that I was naturally generating connection with others and realized that my telling myself 'I am all alone' was not at all true.

If you can be open to sharing, you may find unexpected surprises, new friendships, and quite memorable moments along your way.

What about your career?

Do you have thoughts of doing something slightly different? Or very different? You can change the course of your career and expand in new ways. Ask yourself what you want to be doing and learning about. Explore what matters to you in your career. You can adopt any area of learning that is of interest.

I had recently become a writer about health and disease prevention. I still had my small marketing business. My new passion and career focus was writing. I looked for a fit within the writing and health space and selected a certification course at Harvard Medical School about mind, body, and happiness. Up to Cambridge I went.

There, I met like-minded people who have become lasting friends. This was an exciting fit for me. I was in a historical and unique city, exploring, making new friends, and learning and contributing at a venue I would have never attended in the past.

I joined The New York Academy of Sciences where I attended lectures, conferences, events, and symposia. I met people on the cutting edge of research in all arenas of health. This too held another comfortable new fit with what interested me and what I was up to in life.

You may want another advanced degree. In his 60's, my brother achieved his doctorate. He pursued this due to his own grief. My mother pursued a career in oil painting for 15 years until age 85. It is never too late to dream and to begin working on it.

When you look at your life you may see there are themes of what is important to you. Some people are motivated by the unfairness of politics, some may see that transportation systems need to be altered, and others are always speaking about climate change.

Whatever the interest you have, this may be a good time to take an action toward learning or bettering the world. That may just be the ticket for you to feel better yourself.

In your journal make a list of your current interests, talents, and passions:

- Take a page for each area of life that is important to you to look at what could fit you now. Perhaps include your living situation, family, romantic relationship, friends, hobbies, career, etc.
- Were there dreams you once had but you gave up on? Is it the time to reconsider those?
- Anything can be of interest. You now have a blank slate to write on. There are no rules for what must fit you now. The field is wide open, and you can conjure up anything. For example, you may want to live on a farm or at the beach. You may want to travel or become an artist or musician or perhaps read all the classics.
- There are actions to take to make dreams come true that might fit you now.
- Are there new or resurfaced career goals? Is there interest in training and education needed to reach those goals? Now may be your time.
- What about daily new venues, events, and classes? Are there online, local or distant events or classes of interest? These could be one-off events or a series of classes or even learning to bake bread with a group of friends every week.
- Look at what you might get involved in within your community. There are tons of local organizations in which you could participate

and meet new people while helping others. Make it real.
- Sketch out a weekly plan for yourself. Start by filling up a few time slots for structure upon which to build. For example: dance on Tuesday nights, sketch class on Thursday nights and lunch with friends on Sundays.

Dreams plus actions can equal results!

- Look at what is important to you.
- Tell yourself that your dreams are possible even though you miss your loved one. If you get trapped in the thought that you do not deserve a particular dream or it is not feasible or possible, take one action to pursue that dream right now!
- Do not compare your dream to what you wanted in the past.
- Choose what you want and manifest a great life now.
- Notice that taking action can be very enlivening!

Great work here visualizing a blank canvas and stepping out!

Certain things fit when your loved one was alive and may now no longer fit. In the next chapter we will discuss what does not fit you so that you can see it as freeing rather than experiencing it as a loss.

You've got this.

What Doesn't Fit You

In the end, only three things matter: how much you loved, how gently you lived, and how gracefully you let go of things not meant for you.
BUDDHA

YOUR LIFE HAS CHANGED. There may be things to let go of now that do not fit and don't reflect you. This could be your living situation for starters.

Widows and widowers are warned against making changes within a specific period such as one year after their spouse dies. I recommend that you evaluate your own situation based on what is best for you personally.

Looking back, I wish I had finalized my decision earlier on to qualify for a tax exemption. However, with much effort and wise support, I was eventually able to discern 'what does not fit me now' regarding my living situation and make some unique decisions.

My process went like this:

What doesn't Fit You?

Virtually every morning for one year, I called my dear friend Daryl and we discussed pretty much the same thing. "Should I move or change the apartment and downsize? The space is too big, costly, and too filled with memories."

While I did not want to have the overhead expenses, need all the space or want all the memories, I loved the building, my long-term neighbors, and building staff who were responsive to me which was especially important at the time. There were also elements of the apartment which were rare for New York and convenient with all-inclusive amenities.

I did some fact-finding and looked at another part of the city where I thought I could be happy. The cost was triple what I wanted to spend. I could then hear my late husband in my ear,

> "If you want to be in that neighborhood, stay put and take a taxi over there for breakfast, lunch, and dinner! Hire a limo, even! Knock yourself out! It will be a fraction of what it costs to live there!"

Yes, Tom was super wise and he is always with me. People who die are still with us. We may even 'hear' what they would say in each situation where we think that we do not have the answer.

Having Daryl, a sensible, innovative designer and wonderful listener, was invaluable as I reconsidered my options on an almost daily basis. In the end with her input, I worked out a way to downsize the space that also allowed me to keep half of it.

Do not be rushed by anything if possible. Go at your own pace, and confer with experts who may also care about you.

Does your living situation fit you now?

Do you live in a neighborhood with other couples or young families? Maybe you would like to be away from couple friends? Or you may not be as comfortable living within a community of people with whom you participated as a foursome. Is your current living situation a place for you to flourish, feel comfortable, and at home?

A widow recently shared with me that she kept putting her home on the market and then a few months later after the broker would ramp it up for sale, she would take the apartment off the market. Each time she got close to selling she would visualize bringing everything she owned from her home to her small apartment. Finally, when she closed on the apartment a year later, her broker did not even recognize her reaction. *"Just throw in the furnishings! I just want to be out!"*

There is a readiness to being comfortable with what does not fit you. Again, go at your own pace. You will be ready to take action at some point. Have patience with yourself.

Maybe you would like to live near people who are single and closer to your age range or near family members or friends you love. A widower I know is taking an extended vacation in another country to be with his son and family. He is contemplating what it might be like to live there permanently. This is an excellent idea if you have relatives and want to explore different parts of the world.

You are in a very different situation now and you can consider more clearly where you want to be and what might be a fit for your ideal living situation. You can research this all online and explore synergies in your activities, interests, and tastes in housing.

Right now, I am taking Zoom classes in out-of-town communities which I am 'trying on.' This way I have a chance to hear about living there and meet new people in those areas should I choose to relocate. With a bit of effort, you can explore this as well.

What about your current communities?

Some communities you have belonged to and may have loved may not fit now. You may feel that they do not reflect you or that you are not included in the same way. This could be something you experience especially if the community is couple-based.

In the past you may have volunteered with a group of married women or teams of couples. It might now be time to look at other things of interest and try out new experiences. Approach this openly with fresh eyes. You do not have to desert the communities you have been part of. Just expand. There is a huge world out there when you are open to new things. Adventure, art, music, inspirational venues, communities, learning, etc. You may not yet know what you can find that could be a great fit for you.

I had not known myself to be a dancer, yet in the wake of Tom's death, I've been dancing for a few years now. I am still creating new things in my life I would never pursue if not for my circumstances. Writing this book is an example, and so is learning to play piano.

Give yourself permission. Do not judge yourself about the things that do not fit now. Something enormous has shifted in your world. And perhaps you have sobered more to the finiteness of life. Your interests and needs are different now and you might be expanding yourself as well.

Do the research, find things that catch your eye and interest you. New things might come to mind if you have more time and because of your circumstances.

If that new venue does not work, try something else. There are no mistakes. You are exploring and learning about yourself.

Being Forthright in Relationships

"What do I answer when people ask how I am doing?" one widow asked on Facebook.

Things have changed for you and it does not fit to say you are "fine" when you are not. While you don't have to tell *all*, you can be straight with others. Sharing is powerful. And who knows, maybe they are also dealing with something and you can be mutually supportive and connect in a way that may be different from before.

Embrace Change and Be Open to Listening

People you do not expect might step up to be in your life now. And ones you thought would be there for you may not be, as I mentioned. Have compassion and don't be surprised if some people do not act as you expect. The way you are handling grief may be just fine and it could trigger them, nonetheless. This can sometimes feel unforgivable or hard to imagine, and usually has nothing to do with you.

You might reflect on your ongoing relationships and wonder if they fit you now. For these relationships, you could need to listen *more closely* for their love and caring or you might miss hearing it. (Please, if you like, refer to the chapter 'Staying Connected Regardless of Others' Thoughts' on page 43).

Your people are likely expressing themselves as they usually do, and now you might have a need for more acknowledgment, greater support, deeper involvement, and increased kindness. The same love is likely there.

This is a time to be flexible, open, honest, and to listen closely for the love and connection. Ask for what you need without blaming the other person for not knowing it on their own.

Relationships change because your loved one died. You may want certain people in your life and not others. That is okay. To everything there is a season. As written in Ecclesiastes, there is "a time to cast away stones, and a time to gather stones together; a time to embrace, and a time to refrain from embracing."

Your relationship with your in-laws, despite partner loss, can be deeply rewarding. A widow I know was treated by her in-laws to dinner with her new beau. The beau reciprocated for the holidays. That was indeed a *holiday* miracle for that widow.

Your in-laws' love may present itself in various ways of caring about you. You may be comparing this to how it was before. While things have changed, they have a choice now. And you do too. Relating to them now can be richer for you than ever.

Are you concerned about them? It is their loss too. Are you grateful for them? Can you see that even the smallest things they offer are important? If yes, there is the possibility of having them fit into your new life if you want that and experience the gift that is.

Remember, not everything will fit you now:

- Things that may not fit might include your living situation, communities, hobbies, career, even relationships. And *literally, your clothing may not fit either anymore!*

- As you consider what may not fit now, realize that new situations and people may provide you with something extraordinary that fits well in your current life and there are unlimited possibilities to discover what matters most to you now.
- There is nothing problematic about things or people you enjoyed no longer being a fit. You have had a huge change in your life. And who knows...things and people may fit again later.
- Difficult as it is, attempt to not compare how it was before. This can bring on more distress.
- Be flexible and dream of what could be in your life now.
- Give yourself permission to explore. Be open to where it takes you.

Try this:

Take out your journal and make three columns. Use the categories below or add to it based on your considerations. Write down everything that does not fit and everything that might.

CATEGORY	WHAT DOES NOT FIT?	WHAT MIGHT FIT?
Living situation	My current apartment	Living near family
Relationships		
Hobbies		
Career		
What else?		

Great work! You can now see that certain things fit when your loved one was alive that may no longer fit.

The next chapter is what I discovered about *loving again*. I understood there is no right time to love again. And even more importantly, there is a difference between being ready to love again, accepting someone new, and wanting your spouse back.

The Heaven Can Wait Phenomenon

*I must wait for the sunrise, I must think of a new life,
and I mustn't give in. When the dawn comes,
tonight will be a memory too, and a new day will begin.*
TREVOR NUNN BASED ON THE POEM BY T.S. ELLIOT

SOME PEOPLE RESIGN THEMSELVES to not being open to finding love again. Some people want the love they had previously, and they will not consider anyone else. And some people wonder if they should move forward with romance, and if so, when that might be appropriate.

Regardless of your choice, it is very important to first forgive what happened, to forgive your loved one who died, and to forgive yourself. If you would like to redo the exercises on forgiving, they may provide you with a fresh ability or opening to move forward in choosing a new relationship.

Timing

Many people who do want love again may also have points of view, concerns, and questions about the "right time" to find love in their life again.

The answer is, there is no right time to love again. I have found that when people ask this question, it is because they are thinking about it.

Thinking about it may be a sign that you are ready!

This is your decision alone and there is zero need to explain it or feel shame if it seems too soon or you are worried about what others think. Remember, people will have their thoughts no matter what you decide. Why have someone else's thoughts prevent you from finding love again when you want a relationship?

My First Step: The Ring

The process began with taking my wedding band off. I removed my ring about five months after Tom died when a friend made me aware that I was still wearing it. I had not even thought about removing it. I took it off that week.

It felt odd not wearing it. Vulnerable, too. However, wearing the ring felt untrue. In addition to the beauty of the band of diamonds, I had been placing a significant message on my hand for the world to see: *there is someone in my life loving me, protecting me, being my rock.* Wearing my ring was my way of alerting the world that I still had this love, this rock and protector. Without it, I was just me on my own.

In the wish list letter I wrote that I wanted romance again. I did not realize that I even knew this or could admit this at that time. Perhaps I wanted love again because of the great love I had before. Regardless, I did want love again and though I felt like I had to justify it, I did not.

The Heaven can Wait Phenomenon

Who could you love again?

When your loved one dies, sometimes you seek the same type of person. This is natural to do. However, no one is your late spouse. It is very tempting to choose having someone in your life so that you do not experience the pain of not having your late spouse.

A favorite movie of Tom's and mine was *Heaven Can Wait*.[14] In the movie, a football player named Joe Pendleton, who is very motivated to win the Super Bowl, dies by accident.

Through the magic of cinema, Joe comes back in another's body to fulfill his Super Bowl dream of winning both the game and the girl he left behind. Now inhabiting a new football player's body, Joe, takes Betty's hand saying "It's alright. There's nothing to be afraid of".

Though Betty does not know it is *her* Joe, she says "Your voice sounded so familiar" and portrays sensing the recognition of Joe through expressions of love with her eyes. Without further words, she demonstrates a beautiful, curious, quizzically nuanced recognition of her beloved football player.

Several lines of dialogue moved Tom and I to tears each time we viewed this movie: "I want to memorize everything about you so that no matter what happens I won't forget you. What I am most afraid of is how I would feel if I could not be with you," he says.

And the most poignant line of all, "If you meet a football player someday, you'd give him a chance, wouldn't you?"

---

14 If you have had someone you love die, it is worth seeing this movie and waiting a year or two past their death might be best.

My *Heaven Can Wait* Phenomenon [15]

For me, familiarity and coincidence meant comfort and trust with someone who had associations to my past and similarities to and connections with my late husband, my *football player*.

Within the first year after Tom died, I found myself on long walks or at an occasional movie and dinner with someone I met at a friend's gathering. He was also dealing with the upsetting shock of his wife filing for divorce.

Like my husband, he was a cerebral professional. In fact, he had attended the same specialized, accelerated high school, and early on used the same words my husband had, telling me he was 'a trained observer.' At that year's 9/11 Tribute in Lights, he took me by the hand and pointed up to the sky saying, "Look!" exactly as Tom had done the prior year.

Then came more huge coincidences. I learned that as a young man, he was featured on the cover of a well-known magazine that I recalled reading when I was 21 years old. And of all things, his brother was a crossword editor for that same newspaper. I had recently discovered a pile of his brother's crosswords in Tom's den. Tom had completed dozens of these puzzles over the prior year.

There was kindling for romance, but he was not yet divorced so it ended. This friendship was so related to my past and was indeed a *"Heaven Can Wait Phenomenon."*

About a year later I met another gentleman, a college friend of a friend. He was also smart, a professional, and to his credit and forthrightness,

---

15 The *"Heaven Can Wait Phenomenon"* is my coined term which describes how one can feel attracted to a new partner after their partner dies.

he announced when we met that he was not available. We became friends. We shared the love of music and art, so we casually planned to see the David Bowie exhibit at the Brooklyn Museum.

He was engaging, active, and talented and our commonalities brought us great times. We could laugh and play with words as poetry or song or just be silly and goofy together. He reminded me a lot of my late husband and had a multitude of talents and interests outside his profession. He was a renaissance man like Tom.

Again, more coincidence was that his family and my husband's family were buried yards from each other. He was the same religion as my husband, and of neighboring European descent. Things grew to more than friendship quite organically.

Another *Heaven Can Wait Phenomenon*! Things did not work because there were things of greater urgency to him than romance. I had overlooked that initial *critical piece* he had been so clear about when we first met. Indeed, we did not want the same things from the start. I had only focused on the similarity to my husband and the fun we had. When this ended, I had to look at what drove me to pursue the relationship. I had to admit to myself that I did not want to be on my own nor experience the sadness of being alone. That was what made me so tenacious in having that relationship work out.

The "Heaven Can Wait Phenomenon" can be counter-productive and obscure your view in new romance.

People will likely come into your life and you will compare them to your partner. In others you meet, you may see parts of your loved one's personality; they have a similar profession or hobby or maybe similar kindness, interests, talents or even attended the very same schools. Or maybe they are unlike your late partner and that is a good fit for you now.

I noticed I was explaining to others how like my husband this gentleman was. First, no one really cares. Second, you do not need to justify who you befriend, to yourself nor anyone else. Comparison does occur, yet no one is exactly like your spouse or partner, nor will you ever find someone just like them. Your partner was with you during a specific time in your life. The circumstances of your life are now different. You are different too. Your needs may be different now as well. Maybe you are not looking to have a family with this person or maybe you are. Maybe you want someone to travel with and enjoy companionship and intimacy. Maybe you would rather be with someone who is still working or find someone who is now retired.

Regardless, be aware that comparing this person to your partner who died is likely to leave you and your new partner constrained. You could forgo exploring what may be possible with this new person. Comparison could stop you from appreciating this person for who they are. They will sense this comparison and it will not feel comfortable to either of you. I recommend not comparing anyone to the love you had prior. It is not fun for someone to step into pre-worn shoes.

How to Find Love Again

What I learned from dating after my husband died is that I was not available myself. I wanted love and fun times, and I did not want to be on my own, nor feel the pain of not having Tom anymore. And I realized I was not ready to be in a new relationship just yet.

My love story thoughts always ended with *going off into the sunset hand in hand.* The truth is that no one can come close to meeting your expectations. It is not like years earlier when you meet someone and start a family and start your life together. People may now be at varying stages of their lives, not at the same point.

The ideal way to find love again is to be flexible, happy with your life as it is, and to be interested in getting to know someone for who they really are.

I will find a new partner, but I have given up the idea that I must. I had to discover this on my journey of grief. Yes, I was sad and alone. But I realized I could be okay, even wonderful, on my own. My feeling is that the person you want, not the person you need, will appear when you experience that you are doing well on your own.

I think that if my late husband were watching me, he would be happy about my growth and taken aback that I can navigate the city and boroughs by subway and that I am driving now. I have done some traveling near and far, including other countries like the UK when I made a dream come true and went to Liverpool by myself. I did not do these types of things when he was alive. I have made many strides in my growth and development, and I am living a great life and contributing to others too. In writing this book, I have also been providing more grief expression advocacy work for people whose love ones have died.

In a phrase: I have found myself. Being excited about my life and with who I am today, I am certain I will meet a new man of my dreams for a wonderful future. *And a new day will begin...*

Go at your own pace to love again! Having a new relationship is not a necessity. Certainly you can choose that. Life is for the living and that includes you!

Remember this:

- You are a different person now than when you met your spouse. No one will love you the same way nor have the same history built with you.

- Do not compare people to your spouse who died, even though it is human nature to do that. Being aware of the *"Heaven Can Wait Phenomenon"* as you meet people may remind you that *you do not need any sign of similarity* to your previous love.
- You do not need a 'right' reason to love again, nor anyone's permission about the timing or who you found. *Remember, people will have thoughts, regardless of what you do! You can count on that!*
- You can be patient with yourself and see what you want and what will work best.
- You can create something wonderful with someone if they want something similar to what you want.

We each have the need to connect, to be loved, appreciated, understood, physically touched, and held by others. It is human. We have the need for fun and interesting conversation and exposure to novel things. We need to be stimulated and to stay active. We even need to be making a difference in life.

If you have had wonderful love, or if you have been brave to have had any love, I am confident that you can have love again if you want it.

In the following chapter I will discuss how you can keep your loved one's memory alive for the blessing they were. Honoring them can be very impactful.

Allow yourself to flow with this!

Honoring Your Loved One

*A man does not 'become' what he does.
He brings to his work what he is.*
THOMAS KRANJAC, age 20

MY HUSBAND THOMAS KRANJAC was deeply committed to helping others. There is a stanza in the poem I wrote, *I'm A Grief Surfer*, that reads:

> I will begin to recreate the memory and blessing that my dear Tom was for me and others – the impact of his life and my commitment to carrying the torch for his future memory.

It was instinctive that I wrote this stanza less than two months after he died. I knew in my heart that recreating the memory and the blessing Tom was would allow me to contribute to others in his honor. By keeping Tom's memory alive, I would share what was special about him and manifest that specialness in the world.

Writing this book and helping others with their grief will be perhaps my ultimate tribute to his memory.

Your loved one's memory is a blessing and there are unique and creative ways to keep their memory alive.

Your loved one lived a life. They may have made a difference in the world. They touched others. Having your loved one's life be 'a blessing' is something people say, especially in the Jewish religion. People keep their loved one alive by telling stories about them, by laughing at what their loved one did or said, their *-isms*, and by keeping their words alive by remembering and by sharing them.

I recommend finding unique paths to keep your loved one's memory alive. Consider what they were interested in, passionate about, and involved in. Consider how you can keep the flame of their passion alive in their name.

When my mother died, I made a calendar of her artwork and gave it to people who loved her. Then I gathered 150 of her original oil paintings and presented the collection to The National Museum of American Jewish History at the Smithsonian. Her work was considered for an exhibition there. While no actual show transpired, going through this committee evaluation, and getting her work out to other art history venues made a difference for me in honoring her memory. The Smithsonian gave serious consideration of my mother's artwork and her life — that was a gift to me in helping honor her life as the blessing it was.

My husband was a physician and an artist. I pursued various venues to show his work after he died. I will be selling my mom's and my husband's art and forwarding a percentage of the proceeds to an organization that they might have supported, such as one which supports people with grief, hunger, etc.

Having your loved one's legacy in the mind's eye of others is certainly a way to keep their memory alive. I held two seminars in Tom's honor because he wanted to bring transformational growth and development seminars into the medical field. It was very satisfying to hold events that were well-attended by friends and colleagues who knew and respected him.

Tom had suggested that I approach a public figure, a clergyman, and interview him for a book about his children. After Tom died, I interviewed him three times. He became too busy to complete the book we began but it was a wonderful experience to contribute to my husband's memory, the clergyman, and his family.

It is a common occurrence that people choose a cause to support when their loved one dies. Tom died from sudden cardiac arrest on a tennis court when an ambulance did not come promptly. I worked with the office of Liz Krueger, New York's state senator, to make sure there were AED machines everywhere people were at risk in NYC as there was not one on the tennis court where Tom played that fateful day.

The following year I applied and was retrained in CPR and the use of AEDs (heart defibrillator machines). I then volunteered in the medical tent of the New York City marathon to be there for the health of other athletes in my husband's honor.

My husband's memory that day was top of mind and heart for me. It was an honor to literally 'stand' for the 50,000 runners' health and their triumph over those 26.2 miles. With each athlete who ran past me and with whom I locked eyes and said, "Way to go!" I felt that this profoundly spirit-connected way of serving athletes was an incredible way to keep Tom's memory alive.

What really mattered to your loved one?

What wishes did they want to fulfill? What causes moved them? What would best capture your loved one's memory and legacy to make a difference for others?

This can be a valuable multi-faceted process that can be rewarding for yourself and for the others who remember them, along with those who have been influenced by their work and interests.

Engage with others to honor your loved one:

- Consider everything that was important to them and create a mini legacy around each of those things.
- Look at how disease prevention could have been more present in their life and fashion a way to contribute to others out of the knowledge that is now available to you.
- Use their life to be a full-blown blessing. It likely was. When you take creative action, you honor their memory, make a difference for others, and in doing so you may feel uplifted and connected with them as if they are still alive. *For their memory now is.*

Try this:

- Use your journal and make a list of what projects you may want to create and accomplish. Then take the actions.
- There are unlimited projects and causes that can be acted upon. Do one at a time and keep going.
- You can start now, even if you are sad.

Honoring your Loved One

How great to keep your loved one's legacy honored and alive if you choose to!

In the next chapter we will look at grief and terminal illness and explore how staying connected and communicating during the passages of illness can leave you and your loved one closer and make this difficult time meaningful for you both.

Grief and Terminal Illness

I've seen fire and I've seen rain.
I've seen sunny days that I thought would never end.
I've seen lonely times when I could not find a friend,
but I always thought that I'd see you again.

JAMES TAYLOR
'Fire and Rain'

WE ARE USUALLY NOT READY for someone we love to die. We think we will see them again as the song above goes.

The knowledge that your loved one is terminally ill is extremely sad. Grief begins as soon as you hear of this and continues as you witness their deterioration. There is sadness about their not being able to function, be there for you as they were, the change of the role they played in your life and the sadness you have for them as you consider what they will be missing when they die. You may now even be their caregiver. It is all very sad.

What can you do to have this time with your loved one be precious when it is so awfully sad?

One pitfall of terminal illness is separating yourself emotionally from your dying loved one. It might seem to be the *easy way out,* yet in the end may prove the most difficult to deal with. It is natural for some to want to detach as you might have thoughts to shield your loved one from your sadness about their illness and worries about their death.

Withholding your thoughts, separating yourself and even *faking being positive* to protect them can feel alienating and disingenuous and leave you feeling not so honorable, in addition to being sad.

You *can* choose to continue being connected. You can continue to believe that your presence makes a difference to them even if you think their cognitive challenges are in the way now. This is not about rationalizing what to do, it is about doing what you know is the right thing to do.

You can be genuine. You can share with them appropriately and responsibly how it is for you. You can say things like "I love you; I appreciate you and always have, I wish I could make you all better for you." These are valuable things for you to say if you feel them, even if you think your loved one won't hear or quite understand you. You can also ask them what they want from you now and then see if you can do that.

Be aware that your loved one who is dying, if they have cognitive ability especially, may be grieving as well. They may also now feel that they are *different* from you. They may be comparing themselves to their past level of health. They may be angry, feel no one understands, and that it does not matter anyway.

When my mother-in-law was dying of cancer, I said to her, "Mom we are all dying and some of us just have more details about it. Though it may be sooner for some of us, no one really knows when any of us will die." She said hearing that made her feel better, closer to me, and more a part of life. I have repeated this story to others with apparent terminal illness and it has made a difference. For this is true, we don't know when we will die. No one does.

For someone who has a terminal diagnosis, this window of time to connect may provide you with a chance to repair the relationship with your loved one. Did anything happen between you? If yes, put it right, make amends.

I recall being at my grandmother's deathbed. At 20 years old, I apologized for sometimes having been impatient with her. She lovingly and jokingly said, "Paulette, if you do not stop saying this you will have to leave my room!" Right then I knew she forgave me, and I forgave my impatient self. She died the next day. My relationship with my grandmother was at peace. Nothing was unexpressed nor unforgiven.

Be responsible about what you say and how you say it. Do not be blameful even if you are right. You can say gently what made you angry in the past and that you are expressing it so that there is nothing in the way of expressing your love for them now. Kind communication will make a huge difference in feeling at ease with your loved one during this time. When you reflect later, it will be clear that you used this time together well.

Share everything with fondness so that when you are by their side, there is not a big unspoken emotional boulder in between you both. How you are with them can add to their sense of joy, peace, freedom, calm, and could affect their well-being and their experience of life now for the better.

Writing a letter to your loved one is another useful way to communicate important issues. This is very helpful and freeing as well. You can use it to practice your communication and then choose to say what you need to.

Many people see that at the end of everything, they want to express how much love they have for their loved one. When you get to this point that there is nothing more to say, it is because you said everything that was in the way of your love.[16]

---

16 Paragraph is based on an actual quote, Werner Erhard, *est* Training. "When you've said all the bad things and all of the good things you haven't been saying, you will find that what you've really been withholding is, "I love you."

Another gift you can give your loved one who is dying is to tell them that you will be okay. That you will grieve and be sad and that you will live on and live well. For an infirmed loved one, hearing this can provide a sense of relief, peace of mind, freedom from worry about you and maybe even relieve some of their guilt about dying. Communicating this may free them up to tell you that they want the best for you for a good and fruitful life which could be of much value to you once they die.

In real time, do your best to uphold their medical end of life wishes. They trust you.

It might seem obvious, yet it is important to honor last wishes. Honor the trust they placed in you if you are the holder of the health care proxy and final wishes for your loved one. It is understood and accepted nowadays that when people signed this document, they did not have the *up to the minute* report on the medical advances of those future dates nor the twists and turns of life and death that can occur near the end.

My recommendation is that you abide by the spirit of your loved one's overarching wishes, if not their exact ones. That you make the choice for them with the understanding that medical status in real time is different than a theoretical choice signed at the trust attorney's office. Weigh the choices keeping their preferences foremost at heart.

Do what you think is right. Trust yourself. Perhaps doing what might have seemed 'heroic' then *is* worth the odds. Or perhaps not. Get that second opinion if you need it. Then be gentle with yourself. The same goes with their final resting place if things were left unplanned. They trusted you to carry out their wishes. Doing right by following their wishes as best you can will be freeing for you.

People rationalize end of life decisions claiming that *the deceased or ill person will not know whether their last wishes were carried out*. This is about your word to them and to yourself. Also avoid thoughts of regret and guilt. There is no reason to be plagued with thoughts about how we should have honored them differently. It does matter. Choose to do right by them. Be trustworthy.

Interruptions of grief during your loved one's transition to death.

Once your loved one's death draws near, upset, anger, and blame can emerge. These can be disguises for grief.

You may have been their caregiver or organizer. You became accustomed to this role and routine. Your focus was on those duties. It took a toll on you yet also gave you the sense that you had some control in the process. You had a team. You were in action doing all you could. Expect that there can be a void and that you may feel that you are depressed. This is normal. Stay connected with others and keep sharing your sadness.

Alas, your caregiver role, filled with purpose and action, is ending. You might have thoughts and feelings of having failed. You might blame the hospital, the doctors, a higher power, other caregivers, your loved one, even yourself. This is totally normal.

Forgiveness is in order here. Forgive what everyone did or did not do regarding your loved one's illness and death. This includes yourself, the treatment teams, and your loved one. Then you can just be sad.

For peace of mind:

- Notice you are grieving before your loved one dies.
- Note that your role and theirs has changed and that is sad too.

Grief and Terminal Illness

- If you understand their prognosis and they do not, you can explain it to them. Even though they may not understand, at least be straight with them and be responsible about how you communicate.
- Mainly tell them you love them and what they mean to you.
- Remember we are all dying but no one really knows when or how it will happen. Tell them this. It levels the playing field. It is the truth and a huge gift to them.[17]
- Stay connected to them. It takes one person choosing this – you! Do so even if you do not think they understand what you are saying.
- Communicate anything you want to say before they die to put things right between you both. Either verbally or by letter. Or both.
- Let them know you will be fine and live well. This is a gift to them. They will likely grant you back the wish that they want the best for you in your life.
- Honor their end of life wishes given the reality of their situation.
- Honor their funeral wishes even if these are not your preferences.
- Once they die, be aware that the illness routine ends, and you may grieve for your routinized role in their care. Allow for that and be patient with yourself. Life will pick up and it will pick you up.
- If you blame anyone for something after your loved one dies, write a letter, and forgive whoever and whatever you are blaming.
- Holding onto anger or strong feelings is one way that seems to keep the person alive. However, it does not allow you freedom to be sad or to connect with others.
- Your loved one has died and all that is left is to be sad.

Go easy on yourself. Be sad. Share with others. That is all there is to do. In the next chapter we will discuss sudden death. This is very different from terminal illness.

---

17 *The Needs of the Dying,* David Kessler, 1990.

Sudden Death

Kiss me and smile for me
Tell me that you'll wait for me
Hold me like you'll never let me go
'Cause I'm leavin' on a jet plane
Don't know when I'll be back again
Oh babe, I hate to go.
JOHN DENVER,
'Leaving on a Jet Plane'

GRIEF CAN COME ON SUDDENLY AND SHOCKINGLY. Is grief experienced in the case of sudden death, such as an accident, a suicide, or through an instantaneous life-threatening medical condition the same as grief experienced when someone is dying due to a long-term illness?

Sudden death brings shock which can delay sadness. There seems to be more acute regret and blaming with sudden death than with death caused by long-term illness. I believe more work may need to be done to forgive yourself and your loved one who died suddenly.

Emergencies can cause people to be stunned initially and unable to respond with emotion to what happened. This was my experience. When my husband died suddenly, I did not immediately collapse in tears.

Sudden Death

I was in action doing things I thought I should do. I was calling people. Reaching out to them. I had no personal awareness of hunger or thirst, nor even pain. As I look back, there was no thought about myself nor my needs initially.

I was stunned.

Memories of that day are fragmented. I recall scenes as if I am watching a play.

My hands are on his body and they yell at me, "Don't touch!"

The paddles on my husband at the hospital do not work.

I text one person, "Tom died." I call my cousin and my nephew.

Someone accidentally closes the hospital's automatic door on my finger as I exit. I yell out. Ignoring the pain, I dial my brother in New York.

My son is away at a nearby college. I will deal with that later.

My cousin comes to the hospital. She becomes the 'information hub.'

Next scene takes place in a restaurant with cousins and old mutual friends. They are eating, being jovial, ordering drinks. One has a huge yellow stone on her finger. It is noon.

Making chit-chat, I share about life as if it were still set at 9:19 that Saturday morning, the moment before my life *crashed*.

People order food. I watch them talk and laugh.

I feel physically vulnerable, like I have the flu. I do not want to be anywhere.

New Way to Grieve

I call my son. I tell him by phone. My cousin and her husband and I pick him up at school.

The community begins to gather by my home with food and drink. They are doing things centered around feeding people.

Someone hands me a glass of water. I become dizzy and a doctor friend says I am hyperventilating.

The world is going on around me. People are planning funeral things. I am being asked what I want.

Want. I want to wake up from what seems an unreal nightmare. I want my husband, my rock, my soul mate. Here right now.

I think to myself, "I am totally on my own."

There is arguing among the *funeral planning friends*. The woman with the big yellow stone on her finger has taken over. Everyone has an opinion. I am there watching.

My niece suggests to me that the burial be near the rest of my husband's family. The request has merit. Now I am stressed. I recount that Tom had told me if something happened to do whatever I wanted. I decide to have him buried near my family in another state.

I do not recall most of the people who were in my home nor what they said or did.

Over the next few days, I let out the sadness. I begin to wail.

I do not want to be alone for a moment.

Sudden Death

People come over in droves over a three-day period.

I am told that I should not entertain, just receive consoling.

Services are happening each night in my living room. The initial service is designed to bring my late husband's soul into the space and release it to a higher level. I am not much of a believer in religion but somehow there is a sense of Tom in the midst through the presence of speaking about his deeds, using his words, and my being with our loved ones.

Familiar faces from our entire lives are there at first. People from my childhood, my brothers' friends, our friends during marriage, people from the synagogue.

Chants and hugs happen. One of our old friends touches my back in the gentlest way. I can recall that touch vividly.

Friends are doing household organizing, greeting people, and procuring things for visitors. They bring batches of coffee for themselves and camp out in my home from 9 a.m. to midnight for several days.

It is midnight. I urge them to stay. They leave. I am writing a eulogy at midnight the night before my husband's funeral.

I want my life back. I want to sleep and cry. I want to be left alone. I want to tell the world how wonderful he was. Sharing about his life and his goodness with 300 congregants at the funeral is important to me.

I write for two hours. I am bleary-eyed from tears and uncertain of getting all the details down. I turn in at 2 a.m.

The Funeral

I wear a black dress I bought the week prior. Tom was with me when I bought it. Tom never shopped with me except on vacation. I wonder about the irony of that. Black dress. Bought with him.

My brother from New York steps back into my life for the first time in four years. He literally holds me up at the services.

With family and friends, I begin to feel sad. I cry.

With more relatives at the funeral, more sadness descends.

I notice that it comes in waves. I notice I am shifting from a moment-to-moment unreal theatre into a real sadness.

My brother Larry flies in from California on the redeye and makes it to the services. He drives me, the dog, and two friends to Philadelphia and back. He stays over. My old friend Lydia, who was at our wedding decades prior, stays late into the evening.

Dealing With Life After the First Week

This sudden death threw me into the task of taking care of my son, who was 20 years old and very affected by the sudden loss of his dad – his best friend. As I was grieving, I had to manage my son's suddenly upended life, his well-being, his college career, his health, along with managing my finances, my living situation, and future.

I needed to work through it all and earn money as well.

Some of the work I did then was writing blogs for a public figure about health. Having free choice in subject matter, I chose to research and write about the sudden death of a spouse and its impact on health.

I saw from the literature that a healthy lifestyle for myself could mean a critical difference for my long-range health. With that, I set a course and I chose to meditate rather than medicate, to connect, exercise, eat right, take vitamin D3 and probiotics, get restorative sleep, and to not ingest alcohol.

There was much to deal with logistically. Tom had not prepared for an early death. His personal effects were not in order and he was a collector. He left perhaps five thousand items that I went through, including files and professional records, papers, artwork, documents, artifacts, cameras, rare books, records from his early life, photos, patient charts, clothing, bills, playbills, music, notes, ticket stubs, record albums, and all types of memorabilia and paraphernalia. Everything had to be gone through. It has taken years to accomplish this. And now again, four years after his death, I have called for the storage unit and I am working to downsize the dearer artifacts and the multitude of artwork.

Going through his worldly things of over 67 years was beyond sad and triggering. I am thankful to the few people I hired who helped me box, pack, sort, move, store, shred, and donate. I found having a human being around me was very helpful as so many possessions reflected his artwork, his history throughout our life, and his young life as well as his sentimentality for our times together.

Be aware of traumatic stress. Be easy with yourself.

The amygdala, or the arousal center for brain activity, predicts induced sadness intensity.[18] Though I am not a neuroscientist, I sensed that

---

18 Peter J. Freed, Ted K. Yanagihara, Joy Hirsch, and J. John Mann. *Neural Mechanisms of Grief Regulation*. 27 Feb. 2009. Published online https://doi.org/10.1016/j.biopsych.2009.01.019

my amygdala was very active and susceptible to any strong emotion. I recall a friend saying that when I laughed it sounded like a cry. With awareness, meditation, self-soothing, self-modulating, being on top of your reactions and the impact of them on others, you can handle yourself responsibly. That is what I learned.

For the entire first year I recall having flashbacks of my late husband at the hospital. I was then and for a while, unwilling to hear about a situation or view a movie or play that was anything but loving, happy or humorous. I could not hear about sadness or violence without it triggering my own sadness. Even now, if I hear, read, or see something very sad, I still can experience a wave of sadness that can stay with me a few days.

The work on forgiving myself was very important. And forgiving him. He made decisions that did not turn out well for his health. I did not take stronger actions that might have worked — such as dragging him to the doctor even when he said no. We each did what we did. And we did not do what we did not do. I made peace with all those items and forgave it all.

On Suicide

As I write this chapter on the sudden death of a loved one, I am re-reading a chapter called 'Suicide' authored by my late husband, psychiatrist Thomas Kranjac, M.D. It was published in The Columbia College of Physicians and Surgeons, *Complete Home Guide to Mental Health*.[19]

In the chapter, Tom writes,

---

19 Thomas Kranjac, M.D., a psychiatrist, published in *The Columbia College of Physicians and Surgeons, Complete Home Guide to Mental Health*.

> Following a suicide, the grief and mourning among loved ones can be compounded by anger and self-blame. Some will ask, "How could he or she have done this terrible thing to me?" Others might say, "I drove him or her to it; it's all my fault."

Tom goes on to write,

> These common reactions are based on faulty assumptions in that the majority of people who commit suicide have suffered with depression, alcoholism and other illness before their death and neither they themselves nor their loved ones are responsible for the high level of hopelessness that drove them to take their own lives.

The irony here is that this seems like a personal message to me, though Tom's death was not a suicide. Four years later I uncovered this message directly from Dr. Kranjac to not blame myself. Indeed, this is an important message to discover as I write this chapter.

Takeaways of dealing with sudden death:

- Experiencing grief due to sudden death is different from when terminal illness is present. It can result in a delay of sadness while dealing with your shock.
- Sudden death can lead to more acute blaming of yourself and your loved one.
- Forgiving yourself and your loved one is critical for your future, your dreams, and to be able to take actions to make your dreams come true.
- It is easy to fashion a story around what happened. Just feel the sadness.

- Seek support if you need it to sort out the sadness from the regret and blame. That can be very important for moving forward.
- Seek support to work through the shock and the trauma.
- Be aware of upsetting triggers, avoid them when you can, and be easy on yourself.
- Manage your well-being, including healthy habits. This can serve your future well.
- Meditation can especially help a lot with trauma.[20]
- Utilize the chapter on your well-being while grieving. This can serve your future well.

It was incredibly useful to find this chapter Tom himself wrote. I used it to further take some of the upset away from blaming myself. Life is not always happy nor can we control everything.

Go easy on yourself especially if you have experienced sudden trauma such as this.

This upcoming chapter is about siblings and loss of a parent. It is based on my experience in my nuclear family and what I discovered so that you don't have to endure similar sadness to what I went through.

---

20 Cramer, H., Hall, H., Leach, M. et al. Prevalence, patterns, and predictors of meditation use among US adults: A nationally representative survey. Sci Rep 6, 36760 (2016). https://doi.org/10.1038/srep36760

Creating a Team With Your Siblings
(even if it seems difficult)

You just call on me brother, when you need a hand
We all need somebody to lean on
I just might have a problem that you'll understand
We all need somebody to lean on
Lean on me, when you're not strong
And I'll be your friend
I'll help you carry on
For it won't be long
'Til I'm gonna need
Somebody to lean on
BILL WITHERS
'Lean on Me'

IF YOU HAVE SIBLINGS, YOU CAN PROVIDE EACH OTHER with enormous support and comfort during your parent's illness. And you can be there for each other when your parent dies.

Siblings can rely on each other and take turns caregiving and providing encouragement and suggestions for any difficult decisions. They can share the responsibility at many levels, listening to one another and being a source of kindness and love. Collaborating with siblings can also allow for more creative solutions than handling things on your own may provide.

By sharing stories and laughter about the funny times, poignant recollections, and gratitude for your parents, you keep them alive. Sometimes you may marvel at things you did not know about them but are very happy to learn now through sharing with your siblings. Grieving together can provide a mutual treasure for you and your sibling(s) and help you grieve.

My friend Marge, who has eight siblings, holds Zoom meetings weekly to share these memories, stories, and plans about their lives after their parents died. Through this, they undeniably nurture their own connections and keep their parents' memory alive.

Another friend and his sister manage and utilize their parents' investments to cover the monthly memory support care of their 92-year-old mother. If not for that, both brother and sister would continue to contribute equally to their mother's nursing care. This is teamwork, creative and inspiring.

Being a team with your siblings during times of parental illness and death can be most comforting and reassuring and quite vital for the family's peace of mind. Medical, caregiving support, logistics, and financial decisions for their living situation and treatments are necessary at transitional end-of-life phases for your parents. Sibling collaboration and teamwork for these phases can be a gift within families.

At times even siblings who are not close can find comfort in teaming up at this time. By jump-starting a new and necessary conversation about end-of-life matters, it can also lay a foundation for closeness as siblings confront their own mortality and evaluate their lives and role in the family.

Recent studies have highlighted what may interfere with midlife and older sibling closeness near the end of a parent's life.[21] Such interference, if encountered in your own nuclear family, can feel shocking to you at the time.

Sibling divisiveness is a common phenomenon especially under these conditions:

- The parent is seen as the 'kin keeper' in the family; if they die, a sibling can sometimes step in. And sometimes not.
- When the parent is single, it can put more pressure on the siblings to intervene and cause more strife at times.
- When the parent issues the end-of-life directives to one of the siblings, the other sibling(s) can feel left out.
- The sibling in charge can feel more pressure. Many times, end-of-life directives do not reflect all the medical up-to-the-minute nuances of care. It can be a huge stressor to take on this responsibility by yourself.

This occurred during my mother's end of life. I lived near my mother, seeing her many times a day in various facilities, though she did not assign me as her health care proxy.

There were opinions about her care from one of my brothers who was the health care proxy, though he was not that involved in her hour-to-hour health status. This put much pressure on me and my physician husband to act upon and justify what we perceived and what we suggested.

---

21 Khodyakov, Dmitry, and Deborah Carr. "The Impact of Late-Life Parental Death on Adult Sibling Relationships: Do Parents' Advance Directives Help or Hurt?" *Research on Aging,* U.S. National Library of Medicine, 1 Sept. 2009, www.ncbi.nlm.nih.gov/pmc/articles/PMC2914328/.

From the research it is further noted that regarding siblings: [22]

- It is preferable that the aging parent pick someone neutral outside the family to decide on end-of-life issues.
- In general, sisters are closest with each other during the illness and after the death, followed by brother to brother.
- Brother-sister relationships are not the combination that enjoys the closest relationship outcome.
- When one person seems to do more for the parent, there can be resentment that lasts after the parent dies. This usually occurs when daughters have the principal responsibility for their mothers, and brothers have not stepped up to help.

The process of losing a parent can bring on an added layer of sadness caused by the loss of support of sibling(s) at a time of grief. Though this loss of support may feel like a surprise at that time, the dynamic is somewhat predictable if there has been lifelong favoritism in the family. And remarkably, this may have nothing to do with financial inheritance.

The divisiveness and loss of connection between siblings after losing a parent usually comes out of early family strife, competition, and sibling rivalry that becomes rekindled. Sadness from your parent's death can be more intense when the strife is significant among siblings rooted decades prior and at the core of the nuclear family. Said another way, you may not only lose your parent but also you run a risk of losing sibling(s) in your life after your parent dies.

What may be at play can be attributed to "ancient dynamics" in the family core. This scenario may often be retold as a story, absorbed,

---

22 Khodyakov, Dmitry, and Deborah Carr. "The Impact of Late-Life Parental Death on Adult Sibling Relationships: Do Parents' Advance Directives Help or Hurt?" *Research on Aging*, U.S. National Library of Medicine, 1 Sept. 2009, www.ncbi.nlm.nih.gov/pmc/articles/PMC2914328/.

and inherited almost unconsciously throughout the generations. As siblings growing up together, stories can sometimes be overheard in the background about how this person became the black sheep of their family. In my brother's wife's family, Deborah was 'dead to' her brother. Uncle Jerry had to sneak calls to my mother so that his wife Lil did not hear him converse with his sister.

When I met my 95-year-old aunt whom I had not seen in 60 years, I learned that her mother's brothers were envious of one brother from their country of origin. When this brother gained financial success, the other brothers schemed to burn down his place of business, leaving the brother destitute. I see how this "collective" nattering can be passed down generationally and may not reflect in any way what siblings might gain from the love and support which could be available between them.[23] There were not many stories in my family of loved ones lending a hand, being there to save the day despite all odds, etc. There was not this message in the multigenerational background.

Siblings Can and Do Part Ways After a Parent Dies

Middle-class siblings seem to break away more easily from each other than do working class or poor families. Those from immigrant cultures, especially, often hang together as a way of honoring their parents. Those who do initiate estrangement often feel deep regret later in life.[24]

---

23 Use of the word "collective" with reference to Dr. Carl Jung, that it is in the background of our awareness.
24 Eckel, Sarah, "Why Siblings Sever Ties," *Psychology Today*, 15 Mar. 2015, https://www.psychologytoday.com/us/articles/201503/why-siblings-sever-ties

When dementia is present in the parent, sometimes it compounds underlying sibling issues.

Someone I was providing support to was phoned by the police at 7 a.m. on a Sunday and alerted that her 91-year-old mother was at a train station 200 miles away. The daughter reported this to her siblings and said, "We must do something to help mother. She boarded a train at 5 a.m. and was three days early for the family party!"

The siblings ignored it, thinking their sister was overreacting "*as usual.*" They were in denial about their mother's early morning wandering and dementia. This not only caused fear and worry in the daughter, but sadness to not have her brother's support.

Gossiping and ganging up on the sister, the dynamic in that nuclear family's past, came to the foreground. The daughter was stepping into her lifelong role as the mother's favorite, which brought on more animosity from the older siblings.

The family enlisted help from a social worker. He worked with the siblings and asked the daughter to share her feelings and get help from her brothers, act on it, then report back to her brothers. She agreed to allow any support they could offer and was grateful for their input. When the siblings met together with the professional, everyone was heard, and a treatment plan put into place.

Consider your siblings and the long-term relationship you want with them, way before the illness and death of your parent(s).

- Be gentle with every interaction toward your siblings. Remember that you are each suffering when your parent is sick or dying.

Creating a Team with your Siblings

- Even the sibling who seems preoccupied, abrupt, or short tempered is suffering in their own way.
- Each interaction will be remembered, and you will feel better knowing you treated every family member with respect and kindness when you could.
- If there is strife among siblings, be aware that it may compound the feelings of sadness when losing a parent.
- Stay calm, communicate feelings, enlist friends and professionals to support you during this time.
- Remember you can create a team and can pull together.

You can win individually and as a family. You got this!

In the next chapter, I will discuss how not only holidays and special days, but *anything or anyone* you enjoyed together on any day can be a trigger for grief. I will discuss how to manage this too.

Making It Through Each Day of the Year

Here, making each day of the year
Changing my life with the wave of her hand
Nobody can deny that there's something there.
PAUL MCCARTNEY, CREDITED TO LENNON MCCARTNEY
'Here, There and Everywhere'

THERE ARE THREE TRIGGERS FOR GRIEF. Please be on the lookout. We all know that recalling celebrating special traditions and holidays with your loved one can bring on grief. We also know that nuanced sensory memories, such as hearing their favorite song on the radio, can bring on a spontaneous sadness. I realized too, that the first encounter of being with people who liked or loved my loved one, who miss them and remember them, can also bring on grief.

While you can plan to be with others or do something different on the special days, pop up sensory memories involving music, vistas, etc., can be very triggering in the moment.

And encountering friends and family for the first time after your loved one dies can be extremely sad too.

The sadness does come in waves. I find it very useful to accept that waves will come up. And while I know I will cry or be sad, I also know they will pass.

Grief on Special Days

You have no doubt worried about, read about or experienced already, how the first holiday, the first New Year's, the first wedding anniversary, the first birthday will be.

You can prepare for these special days and set things up to not be alone. If possible be with someone who cares about you. Attempt to make the day special in a *different* way. This takes some purposeful planning on your part and perhaps telling others what you are doing so that they can support you or be with you then if you want their company. You might also carve out a time and place to honor your loved one's memory on that day.

I have a new tradition with a widow friend who asked me to have dinner with her near my birth date so that she can celebrate with me and make a new memory for herself as that is near the date her husband died. For three years now we have created a new memory and celebration together, always at a fine steak restaurant. I am happy to make that a fun evening for her when it could be a sad time if she were alone. And I get to share my birthday with my friend, enrich the friendship, continue a *new* tradition, and get the chance to eat some very fine steak in the process.

Grief Brought About Through Nuanced Sensory Memories

Not only may traditional days bring on memories but so can the simplest sensory experiences that you shared with your loved one. Your day-to-day life can bring about these vivid nuanced memories that usually appear suddenly and unexpectedly. Anticipating that *waves* of grief come up may be a useful paradigm to hold, as well as the knowledge that you can get through the sadness.

About two years after Tom died, someone turned on a radio and the calypso style song *Somewhere Over the Rainbow* made for Pixar's short film *Lava* came on. Tom and I had seen that short about a year before he died.

It is a love story about two volcanoes; an older man volcano seeking love sings the rainbow song to a younger female volcano. She does not respond to his song. Experiencing extreme loneliness and heartbreak for his unrequited love, he begins to wither and die. Just in the nick of time he hears the younger female volcano singing his song back to him and his fire reignites, saving his volcano life as they become one single island. Tom sobbed during this short movie.

Now it was my turn. I excused myself speedily to the restroom, stopped the volunteer work I was doing, and I had quite a forceful cry. A few moments later, I joined back in with the cause. *This is surfing the mightier waves.*

Examples of Nuanced Sensory Memories

A storm you are now weathering alone resembles one you rode out 'huddling and cuddling' together; the vibrance of an early morning sunrise evokes your last trip walking hand in hand on the beach; a season changes and the promise the new one holds takes you back; a delicious platter of food set before you has you missing the enjoyment of wonderful meals together. Fragrance inhaled on someone walking by, the softness of a scarf you touched, a flower's color in springtime, a familiar street you rarely walk down yet they loved. Passing your favorite restaurant shared for only special times, seeing a ball game with their favorite team, hearing the music theme of their favorite show, recalling the closing song they always played on guitar in their nightly serenade to you, passing the place you first kissed, election day voting when in complete surprise, you see their signature from four years ago.

You may recall your loved one and being with them in each of these contexts. The slightest sensory recall of touch, sight, taste, smell, and sound can have you reliving these memories, bringing on sadness and tears. Experience the sadness which can tend to hit unexpectedly. Keep going. The sadness will fade.

Share the stories provoked by these sensory recalls as you keep their memory alive. Be cautioned as you retell the story of a particular event in the past to not finish the story with, "I will never be as happy again." Merely share what happened and allow yourself to experience the sadness if it comes.

Honor the day or nuanced memory with time alone. Honor it with others who remember her/him too. Honor it by planting a tree in their name, by saying a prayer, by lighting a candle, by holding a fundraiser gala with their artwork and giving the proceeds to a cause they loved. Honor them by continuing to make their life a blessing through things that are important to you and what you think would be important to them.

People Who Were Close to Your Loved One

You may see your loved one in their memory or in their twinkling eye. You may experience your loved one in their kind words about them or you may feel your loved one's presence in their hug.

For me, sadness comes any time I meet someone who I have not seen since Tom died. Being with them I experience who my husband was for them in their life. It is like Tom is *alive* again for that split second. I then feel sad for that person and who Tom was for them and for myself missing Tom. Maybe that is the same for you as well.

Leaving folk dance one night almost four years after Tom died, I ran into a fellow parent, a dad, and his two grown sons who used to play with my son when the kids were eight years old. As parents we used to do things together, too. I had not seen them in at least ten years. They knew about my husband's death and uttered very kind words. Tom was *alive* again for a moment and I felt the love they had for him and the compassion for me. No sooner did I leave the elevator we rode together that I noticed tears were coming fast out of my eyes.

Making it through each day of the year:

- Prepare for special traditional days and do not be alone if possible. Do something new to make a new memory.
- Honor your loved one's memory on that day if you like as well.
- Nuanced sensory memories can make grief appear suddenly and unexpectedly. Be aware of this possibility and make room for possible sadness. Then *surf* it.
- Beware that sadness can come suddenly, especially the first time you encounter someone who cared about your loved one. There is

no time limit on this. Even if it is years, you may still react to their love for your loved one.
- Realize that it is wonderful that you had your loved one in your life and wonderful that you keep their memory alive.

This is part of life. And it is very wonderful that you can experience your love for your loved one. You are doing just fine.

In the next chapter I will detail how living your purpose can make for a powerful life!

Living Your Purpose

First when there's nothing
But a slow glowing dream
That your fear seems to hide
Deep inside your mind
All alone I have cried
Silent tears full of pride
In a world made of steel
Made of stone
Well, I hear the music
Close my eyes, feel the rhythm
Wrap around
Take a hold of my heart
What a feeling
Bein's believin'
I can have it all
Now I'm dancing for my life
DEAN PITCHFORD
'What a Feeling'

THE LAST STANZA OF THIS QUOTE ABOVE, yes, what can *take hold* of *your* heart?

I suggested earlier in the book that you make a list of what you dream about and open it six months later. When you open that letter, you may be surprised with what you wanted for yourself — even early on after your loved one died. Perhaps you have considered things that might *fit you now*. You may have dreams and wishes for yourself and your family as you always did, and you wonder what your purpose in life really is especially now that your loved one has died.

For some of us it is obvious. Even in our sadness, we do want to live on and be happy and healthy. We want the same for our loved ones, our communities, and we have the highest hopes for the world at large.

One significant thing I learned from my grief journey is that acting on what matters to you is a powerful thing you can do in moving forward with life. You will be shifting your thoughts away from yourself and toward something more important perhaps. You may very well already know what makes a difference to you and what got you out of bed in the morning, especially before your loved one died and before your grieving. You may already have and espouse that purpose in your life.

My journey of extreme sadness culminated in writing this book and in supporting others who have had a loved one die. My path revealed a new way to grieve. I am committed to share my journey so that people understand that they have a choice in how to grieve. That they do not have to have a grim future of sayings and thoughts such as, "It is over for me!" or, "It is never going to work out!" Or even that the best thing to do is to 'keep busy.'

Perhaps look at your future from the vista of that which is important to you. Look at how you can see yourself emerging as someone who might want to share something based on something you know, have nurtured, or even based on something which *irks* you that you would like to see *put right*. Look at this from the standpoint of what you might like to contribute to others. You need not formulate how this might occur. Just look at what you think about, what you read about, what issues you involve yourself with. Look at what people know about you and what you speak to them about.

Over time I have sought to make a difference with my knowledge. I researched and discussed health and prevention and created a short, simple PowerPoint video with the world's expert on vitamin D, called The ABCs of Vitamin D.

I wanted to help others' health from a prevention standpoint. And as a marketing executive, I wrote about cause marketing (the positive impact of brands contributing to a cause). I have written about alternative forms of advertising, such as inserts placed into outgoing shipments of mailed merchandise and unconsidered revenue for direct marketing brands doing that. Things in life have mattered to me and I saw them as avenues in which I could make a difference.

After Tom died, and once I was clear about what was important to me, I took actions. His death made it of utmost clarity that defibrillators should be anywhere human beings were at risk. I set a course to make sure that this would happen throughout New York City. I did this to honor Tom's memory. I felt empowered by having something in my life that had meaning to me, something that might someday matter to others too. I did not want anyone else to die because a defibrillator was not in a place where people exercised and might be at risk.

Once you are clear about what matters to you, get involved and take actions to make the world a better place around that issue. You can get involved on a small scale or a very large scale.

Your purpose in life is yours and it can evolve.

Living your Purpose

To summarize:

- By taking on what matters to you and living your purpose, you can experience real power and joy.
- You can move you forward in your life, standing for what is important, and you may be doing good for others well.
- Acting on that which matters to you is perhaps the most wonderful culmination of your grief journey. You will be shifting your thoughts away from you and toward something even more important.
- To find your purpose, look at what matters to you, what you complain about, what irks you, and maybe what you have some knowledge about.
- See what you might do to make the world a little better in this area. Do not give up if you cannot save the whole world. He who saves one person does save the world.[25]
- Living your purpose can also help you connect with others. Others may participate with you, be moved, and inspired by you, may act on their own or may even become your fans and cheer you on.
- Be powerful. Step out. Express yourself and your ideas. You have wisdom. You are alive.

Just do it!

In the final chapter, I will share about what I am planning next. I hope you will try on what is next for you as well.

---

25 *Babylonian Talmud*

What Is Next?

Things are things, they can be replaced. People cannot be.
SYLVIA TUNIS, MY MOTHER

THE PHRASE 'THINGS ARE THINGS' became a mantra to me. If a precious thing broke or got destroyed, if a piece of jewelry broke or was lost, my mom's words always served to reassure me. I recall when my business took a downturn in 2007, my mom so wisely stated, "Paulette you are the same person, do it again!"

Many people whom I loved and was close to died within a short time period. I can never replace my mom, my husband, my in-laws including my brother-in-law Anthony and his parents, my nephews Michael and Stephan, great aunt Billie and her adult children, my cousins Wesley and Mickey, etc.

Some of those who died were the closest, the strongest support, the ones most committed to me and my life, the most loving, the wisest and kindest, the ones that were always there and had my back and to whom I could always turn. They were wonderful relatives and exemplary family members.

Tom's and my world, which had begun with such abundance and love, had shrunk so much in one decade to become 'just us' with each person who died and each divorce and move that occurred.

What is Next?

Tom would hold me in his arms and say, "We have each other and it's now 30...41½, 43½ years."

And suddenly we did not have each other. I did not have someone dedicated to having my back regularly, lovingly, supportively, immediately, wisely, brilliantly, and committedly. I missed my husband and being able to share our joys, our sorrows, and our days. I missed having someone who cared so much about what I was up to.

When I was growing up and building my life, there were abundant connections with people, more with every decade. Since the death of my mother and then my husband, a sizable discovery for me is that I will never take any interaction for granted. I consider an invitation to anything as a wonderful opportunity and never a given. I attempt to honor people having a place in my life even if they are not who I choose to be with 100% of the time. I consider anyone wanting to know me and include me as a gift.

There are tons of amazing people with whom to connect. I have connected with so many. I know from when my husband died and when my mom died just four years prior that every moment in my life is a creation.

I have walked New York City as *A Grief Surfer* — crying when I left a venue, especially.

It hits me to this day. I miss Tom. I miss being a partner and having a partner. I miss the identity of being a wife, the honor of being a respected doctor's wife, having a hearth and a moment-by-moment relationship like I had. I was cherished by him, starting in my late teens. We shared and built our lives and reached for the stars and the future together. I will not know that exact type of relationship again.

That is what my mom meant; you cannot replace people.

As *A Grief Surfer*, I frequently separate out the ridiculous thoughts popping up in my head that it is 'just me' and 'I won't be happy again' or 'I have to brave life alone' or some variation on that theme.

No one will be Tom. And they are not my mom, either.

Though I cannot replace people, people are unique and wonderful.

New people have been there for me and I for them. Maybe not exactly as it was with the incredible people who died. Yet, people have been there for me with love, immediacy, and unthinkable support. People have had my back too.

My life is great and miraculous.

I have created several communities of people that I now know as 'family.' I have discovered that I am a dancer, and that dancing brings me joy.

I have become a better parent for my son. We have grieved. We have been welcomed at many other family tables for holidays. I have earned my real estate license and become an expeditor. I have downsized and have become debt-free. I am raring to be on the next lap of this continued journey called life.

The most significant thing to come out of the deaths I have encountered is that I have realized my purposes in life. I have been doing grief expression advocacy work to help people manage grief which has culminated in my writing this book. I am planning to help more people with their grief based on what I have learned myself.

What is Next?

I will be providing more interaction on my website:

www.newwaytogrieve.com

I would be honored to have you share this book with your friends and family and follow me at:
www.facebook.com/newwaytogrieve
www.instagram.com/newwaytogrieve
www.twitter.com/newwaytogrieve

Recently reviewing some of Tom's artwork, I have located historical art shows in which his art appeared. I am committed to giving his diverse, creative, colorful, and beautiful work a rightful place in art history. From an early Masbeth Peace Festival in 1970 where his small peace 'posters' were featured with Ad Reinhardt's, Mark di Suvero's and Robert Rauschenberg's works to a Fiftieth Anniversary Show at Terrain Gallery in NYC in 2005 where his work was shown with Robert Motherwell's art, it will be an honor to make Tom Kranjac's work available, give a portion of the sales towards grief supportive organizations and share the story of his journey and his influencers.

I was able to show the famous and late Ivan Karp (2005 or so) Tom's portfolio at Okay Harris Gallery in NYC. He commented that Tom's use of color was extraordinary and that the work portrayed an artist replete with wholesome openness, goodness and generosity.

Yes, that was Tom Kranjac. As artist, as physician, as husband, father and as man.

Since these early days of grief surfing, I continue to create new relationships and pursue things in which I am interested. And make a difference for others.

Mom, you were right: you cannot replace people. They will be in our memories forever.

And:

- You can have people in your life for whom you matter and who matter to you. You can always have this.
- You can build and rebuild your dreams.
- You can welcome wonderful, loving, and caring people into your life. The world is filled with them.
- No one can replace your loved one.
- You can indeed accomplish feeling very loved and enriched by others in many ways you never dreamed possible.

I promise.

Acknowledgments

Profound thanks to my coach Armand DiCarlo with whom I discovered that writing and making this book accessible to people who grieve (so that they do not have to suffer more because of their added thoughts and worries) is part of what I experience as a blessing for my future and my work.

Tremendous gratitude to Werner Erhard whose work of transformation has allowed me to create the following: a remarkable marriage with the man of my dreams, completion of my master's degree at age 25 after doing the *est* Training, a successful, enduring marketing business based on providing significant results for corporations. The 'distinctions' from this transformational work have allowed me to powerfully keep going, generate my life regardless of my circumstances, and share with others. This book is the culmination of my journey.

To my oldest brother Larry, who shared transformational education with me in 1978, who has "had my back" since birth, and who has been an incredible inspiration and beacon of how to be and function through life's transitions, progressions, and grief.

Acknowledgement to my internist of 30 years, Alex Sherman, MD, who, during lockdowns of COVID-19, was there by video being supportive of my well-being, reassuring my efforts of writing this book, and cheering me on.

To friends who took the time to read this book in its earlier stages and provide helpful feedback: Diana Cretella, Ninel Kandova, and Robert Stern, MD.

To the extraordinary people along my journey who not only 'saved the day that day' by steadying me on my surfboard, but who provided the ultimate gift by showing me that I could still ride.

In no significant order they are:
Marge Carney, Nana Greller, Donna Landa, Shelley, Jeffrey and Isabel Cahn, Diane Weiss, Rabbi David Ingber, Luis Marcos MD, Norman Rosenthal MD, Bob Roth, Cindy Lauda, Fran Beallor, Rich Kranjac, Liz Kranjac, Anna Olivero MD, Steven Kaplan MD, Steven Weinstein MD, Douglas Moss MD, Reverend Eleanor Bregman, Dane Kranjac, Adriana Kranjac, Glenn Jacobi, Howard Tear, Jane Tear, Douglas Moss MD, Russell Berdoff MD, Fred Kass MD, Neill S. Cohen Psy.D, Daryl Pines, Michel Obadia, Lory Gitter, Steve Walter, Foroogh and Shoray Zarinehbaf, Amy Wilkins, Betty Bianci, Meredith and Steve Wolfe, Elle Jackson, Jo Blackwell Preston, Kathy Torrey, Richard Rosen, Laurie Landa, Kristin Meade, Jane Martin, Shir Yaacov Feit, Jamie Askin, Robert Tunis, Stefanie Rennert, Ashley Henry, Tami Zackrie, Laurie Langer, Jonathan Meyer, John Kranjac, Emily and Dan Adler, Ellen Warner, Ruth Goodman, Marsha Meislin, Suellen Carney, Mark Podwal MD, Basya Schecter, Tara Kutsi, Ann Marks, Ken Abelson, Ariela Noy, Bob Meyers, Phyllis Dubrow, Anthony Barrett, John Zambetti MD, Philip Diperna, Nick Agneta, the late Ellen Fine Levine, Adina Zion, Evan Torgan, Santos Vargas, Keith Torgan, Barbara Siesel, Denise Jackrel, Joseph Rosenthal, Ya'el Chaikind, Scott Epstein, Dan Gluck, Annette Friend, Susan Knapp, Lydia Burdick, the late Richard Ambrosio, Eric Teitel MD, Ken Malek, Charles Clement, Larry Pearson, Rosemarie Barrett, Gary Thompson, Mario Iturbides, Fran Harris, Steve and Sharon Bajada, Michel Obadia, Lois Hall, Dr. Sherry Schecter, Michael and Josselyne-Herman Saccio, Valerie Barnard Kanofsky and Marla Alt.

Acknowledgements

To Facebook groups of widows and widowers who 'hearted' my answers by the dozens, showing me I have a song to sing for people who have had their loved ones die.

To Brian Kurtz, an extraordinary health marketer and writer whom I have known over decades, who took this book seriously and provided me with a talented editor.

To Molly Pearson, a thoughtful, artful, sprightly, and responsive quality editor, who, like a better tennis player in rally, helped me to 'up' my author 'game.'

I thank you all. From the bottom of my heart.

Paulette Kranjac

About the Author

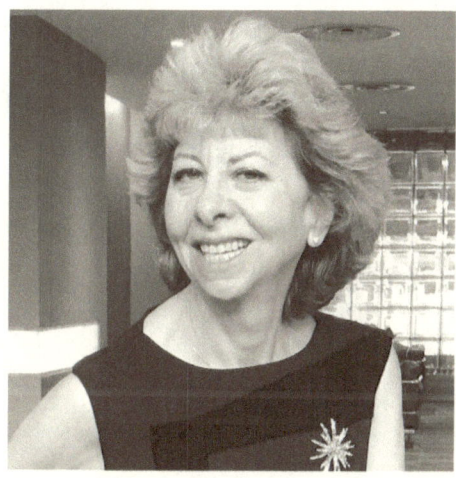

Paulette Kranjac's *New Way to Grieve* came about due to her substantial losses in a short period of time. Those led to a personal discovery about grieving which she is committed to sharing with others. Her mission is that people whose loved ones have died do not have to experience unnecessary suffering and pain. She has supported many people whose loved ones have died.

Paulette has been a marketing entrepreneur for four decades and has worked with large mail order catalog businesses to significantly increase their number of customers. Paulette has done web design, been a content writer for a physician and public figure, a health writer, an informed health advocate and coach.

She was honored by the Direct Marketing Association in 2007 for her contributions in marketing. More recently, she obtained her real estate license and license as a permit filing representative specifically to assist those who want to move or structurally change their homes after the death of a loved one.

About the Author

Paulette has a Master's degree in psychology from CUNY Hunter College and is actively working with people whose loved ones have died, as a Grief Expression Advocate, as time permits.

A longtime athlete, Paulette has been working out for 43 years and folk dancing for the past three. She lives in New York City with her 13-year-old Shih Tzu, Sandi.

You can reach her at pkranjac@newwaytogrieve.com.

About the Cover Art

Seascape Number 1, acrylic (January, 2009), Tom Kranjac.

Tom was a psychiatrist and psychoanalyst as well as an abstract impressionist and contemporary artist. The cover reflects the 'surfing' of grief, the waves that we survivors ride.

It is an honor to incorporate Tom's artwork in conjunction with this book.

Cover design by Steve Funaro.

www.ingramcontent.com/pod-product-compliance
Lightning Source LLC
Chambersburg PA
CBHW021954290426
44108CB00012B/1072